I0569665

Worry Is a Waste of Your Imagination

Strategies for a Worry-Free Life

Joanne Harvey MSW

Copyright © Joanne Harvey 2024. All rights reserved

eBook ISBN: 979-8-9919970-1-0

Paperback ISBN: 979-8-9919970-0-3

No portion of this book may be reproduced, distributed, or transmitted in any form or by any means—through photocopying, recording, or other electronic or mechanical methods—without the author's express written consent. Exceptions are granted only for brief quotations used in critical reviews or other noncommercial purposes as copyright law allows. For permission requests, please get in touch with the publisher at Joanne Harvey

The names, personal details, and identifying characteristics of individuals mentioned in this book have been changed to protect their privacy. Any resemblance to actual persons, living or deceased, is purely coincidental. The stories and case studies are based on real experiences but have been modified to ensure anonymity and confidentiality.

DISCLAIMER

The information in this book, 'Worry is a Waste of Your Imagination: Strategies for a Worry-Free Life,' is based on the author's personal experiences, research, and insights. It provides a reliable resource for your journey to a worry-free life.

The techniques and strategies discussed are meant to support personal growth and well-being but may not be suitable for everyone. If you have a medical or psychological condition, please seek advice from a licensed healthcare provider before implementing any techniques or exercises mentioned in this book.

The author and publisher disclaim any liability for any direct or indirect consequences arising from the use of or reliance on the information contained in this book. The reader assumes full responsibility for their actions and decisions and should exercise caution and discretion when applying the practices discussed.

By reading this book, you agree to take full responsibility for your well-being and acknowledge that any reliance on the information provided is at your own risk.

Contents

Acknowledgments

To my dearest husband, you are my rock, biggest supporter, most enthusiastic cheering section, and truest confidant. Your unwavering belief in me and your constant encouragement have made all the difference in my life.

This book is as much yours as it is mine. Your insights, support, and patience have been invaluable in shaping this journey. Thank you for walking beside me, for the countless conversations, and for always reminding me of what is possible. Your presence fills my heart with joy and my life with meaning.

***

To my incredible clients, who have come to me burdened with anxiety and worry, you are the true heroes of this journey. Your courage to face your fears, confront your worries head-on, and commit to the hard work of recovery is nothing short of inspiring. It takes immense bravery to seek help and even more to stay the course when the path is challenging. Your determination is a testament to your strength.

I am profoundly grateful for each of you—your trust in me, your willingness to be vulnerable, and your openness to share your experiences. Your stories of struggle and resilience have taught me so much about the strength of the human spirit. You have shown me that recovery is not just about finding relief from anxiety but about rediscovering hope, joy, and the possibility of a brighter, more fulfilling life.

Thank you for allowing me to be a part of your healing journey. Your progress and recovery are a testament to your determination, and I am honored to have witnessed your growth. Your journeys have not only transformed your lives but have also deeply enriched mine. Because of you, I continue to be inspired daily to do this work, and I am grateful for the opportunity to learn from your experiences.

With deep gratitude and respect,
Joanne

Introduction

The Contradiction of Worry

Worry often feels like a necessary part of life. It can seem as though by worrying, we are preparing ourselves for potential dangers or preventing future problems. However, worry is more often a thief than a friend, stealing away our present peace and joy. For many of us, life's constant demands—balancing work, family, finances, and personal well-being—can turn worry into a habit that feels impossible to break.

But what if we could change our relationship with worry? What if we could learn to use the same mental energy spent on worry to imagine positive outcomes, dream big dreams, and live more creatively? This book is designed to help you make that shift. It provides practical tools, exercises, and real-life stories to demonstrate how to transform worry into a catalyst for growth, creativity, and peace.

Worry is a waste of your imagination,
and it was written for you.

This book is tailored for adults who find themselves trapped in cycles of worry. Whether about children's futures, aging parents, health concerns, financial stability, career transitions, or the state of the world and so many other subjects, this book offers strategies to help you move forward. Worry often feels productive, but it keeps us stuck in fear. I aim to help you transition from a fear-driven mindset to one filled with hope, resilience, and creativity.

The Purpose of the Book

"Worry is a Waste of Your Imagination " offers a roadmap to help you navigate the maze of worry. I will explore the nature of worry and how it impacts your mind and body and provide actionable strategies such as mindfulness, cognitive restructuring, emotional resilience-building, and imaginative exercises. With a blend of scientific insights, practical exercises, and inspiring stories, you will be empowered to reclaim your mental space for positive, creative thought.

I hope this book teaches you how to replace worry with mindfulness practices, cognitive behavioral techniques, emotional resilience strategies, healthy habits, and supportive relationships. By the end of this journey, you will be equipped with a comprehensive toolkit to live a worry-free, imaginative, and fulfilling life.

"Worry does not empty tomorrow of its sorrow.
It empties today of its strength."

— CORRIE TEN BOOM

Chapter 1

The Nature of Worry

What is Worry?

Worry is an emotional state characterized by anxious thoughts about potential future events. It is essentially the mind's attempt to foresee and prevent problems before they happen. While a certain level of worry can be expected and even helpful in small doses—like when preparing for an important presentation or planning a family trip—chronic worry is different. Chronic worry is a persistent state of anxiety that keeps us stuck in a loop of negative thinking, often without resolution.

The Difference Between Worry and Concern

Concern is grounded in reality and typically prompts constructive action. For example, feeling concerned about your child's performance in school may lead you to talk to their teacher or help them with homework. Worry, conversely, is more speculative and often involves imagining worst-case scenarios that may never occur. Concern leads to problem-solving, while worry keeps us stuck in a cycle of fear and anxiety without taking action.

Common Sources of Worry

We often experience worry related to several key areas:

Health and Aging: As we age, the natural changes in our bodies can become a significant source of worry. The awareness of physical decline, the onset of chronic conditions, or the potential for sudden illnesses can overshadow daily life. For some, the loss of mobility or cognitive function becomes a daunting prospect, leading to fears about losing independence or becoming a burden to loved ones. This worry can be exacerbated by seeing peers or older family members go through similar experiences. Moreover, the media often highlights diseases associated with aging, such as Alzheimer's or Parkinson's, further intensifying these concerns. Worries about health aren't just about the physical aspects but also the emotional and psychological toll of aging, grappling with the reality of one's mortality.

Family and Relationships: Our roles within the family continuously shift, bringing new challenges and worries at each stage. Raising children presents its own worries, from concerns about infant safety and developmental milestones to worries about adolescent behavior, teenage rebellion, and the decisions young adults make as they step into independence. Parents often grapple with fears about their children's futures, wondering if they will find stable careers, maintain healthy relationships, or fall into pitfalls like addiction or financial trouble. The possibility of children making poor life choices or facing mental health issues adds layers of concern.

An excruciating challenge is the distance or estrangement that can develop between parents and their adult children. This separation might be due to physical distance or emotional divides caused by unresolved conflicts, differing life choices, or misunderstandings.

The reasons are often complex, from lifestyle disagreements to deeper feelings of betrayal or hurt. This estrangement can leave a profound sense of loss, helplessness, and a longing for connection, creating a void that is hard to fill and leading to persistent feelings of grief and anxiety.

In addition to worries about our children, many find themselves taking on the role of caregiver to aging parents, which comes with its own set of stressors. Concerns about providing adequate care, the emotional toll of watching a loved one decline, and balancing caregiving with personal and professional responsibilities can be overwhelming. There may also be guilt or tension with siblings over caregiving roles, further complicating family dynamics.

Midlife often brings relationship challenges within marriage or partnerships. As couples face an "empty nest," underlying issues may surface, revealing strains previously masked by the busyness of family life. Differing views on retirement, leisure, and future goals can create friction. Additionally, fears around aging and the potential loss of a partner, whether through emotional disconnection, divorce, or death, can heighten anxiety.

Worrying About Finding a Life Partner. Are you caught in the cycle of worrying about finding a life partner? It's a common fear that many of us share. The mind often races with thoughts like, *"What if I never meet the right person?"* or *"What if I'm meant to be alone?"* These worries can feel overwhelming, especially when society emphasizes relationships as a measure of happiness and success.

But here's the thing: worry is a waste of your imagination. It tricks you into believing you must predict the future or control every outcome to find fulfillment. Worrying doesn't bring you closer to your future partner; it only drains your energy and limits your joy in the present moment.

Instead of getting lost in the what-ifs, imagine a life filled with love, whether it comes from a partner, friendships, or self-love. Trust that the journey to finding a life partner doesn't have to be filled with anxiety and fear. It can be a beautiful exploration of who you are and what you want. By letting go of the worry, you open yourself to life's endless possibilities.

Remember, the energy you spend worrying could be better used dreaming, creating, and embracing the life you have now. Trust in the process, be open to new experiences, and know that the right person will come into your life at the right time.

Financial Security: Financial concerns can strike at any stage of life, each bringing its own set of worries. In early adulthood, there is often anxiety over student loans, finding a stable job, and building a foundation for financial independence. As we move into our middle years, worries shift towards managing mortgages, rising living costs, and saving for children's education—all while trying to prepare for retirement—the fear of not having enough saved, unexpected medical expenses, or job insecurity can create significant stress. Later in life, concerns about outliving savings, maintaining a comfortable lifestyle on a fixed income, or dealing with unforeseen expenses like long-term care can weigh heavily. Each phase brings its financial challenges, often leaving us questioning if we're doing enough to secure our future.

Career Transitions: Career transitions can strike at any age, shaking the very foundation of our identity and sense of purpose. In midlife, these changes often feel particularly seismic—whether driven by personal choice, economic upheaval, or sudden organizational shifts. The fear of being pushed out, becoming irrelevant, or needing to pivot to an entirely new path can create a whirlwind of anxiety. But it's not just about holding onto a job; it's about finding meaning and fulfillment in what we do. The challenge of redefining oneself, learning new skills, or proving one's worth again can feel daunting, leaving many questioning their future, their value, and their place in a rapidly changing world. These moments demand courage and resilience, pushing us to adapt, reinvent, and ultimately discover new opportunities in the face of uncertainty. And can cause hours of worry.

Mortality and Legacy: Death can touch our lives at any age, often catching us off guard with its suddenness or inevitability. When a friend or peer passes away—whether unexpectedly or from a terminal illness—it can hit close to home, stirring deep worries about our mortality. It's a stark reminder of life's fragility and unpredictability. As we grow older, these thoughts can intensify, leading us to reflect on our remaining time and the legacy we hope to leave behind. We may wonder how we'll be remembered or if our lives have made a meaningful impact. This existential worry isn't just about the fear of death but a more profound concern about having truly lived, loved, and left something worthwhile behind. Such reflections can be unsettling but also a call to embrace life more fully, cherish our connections, and make the most of the moments we have.

> *"Worrying is like paying a debt you don't owe."*
>
> — MARK TWAIN

The Cost of Chronic Worry

Chronic worry exacts a significant cost, often creeping into every aspect of life and silently wearing down both the body and mind. Physically, the body responds to prolonged stress by staying alert, frequently called the "fight or flight" mode. This constant state of vigilance can lead to various physical symptoms, such as persistent headaches caused by muscle tension in the neck and shoulders or even migraines triggered by stress. The constant release of stress hormones, like cortisol, can raise blood pressure, putting undue strain on the heart and increasing the risk of cardiovascular diseases. Digestive issues, such as acid reflux, irritable bowel syndrome, or stomach ulcers, can also arise from the body's stress response, as chronic worry disrupts normal digestive functions. Moreover, prolonged stress can weaken the immune system, making the body more susceptible to infections and illnesses and slowing recovery from sickness.

Mentally, chronic worry can be equally debilitating. The constant barrage of anxious thoughts can lead to overwhelming fatigue as the mind is perpetually engaged in overthinking and scenario-building. This mental exhaustion often spills over into emotional regulation, making individuals more irritable or prone to mood swings. Sleep disturbances, such as insomnia or restless sleep, are common, as worries play on a loop in the mind, preventing restful sleep and leading to a vicious cycle of exhaustion and anxiety. Over time, this relentless mental strain can develop into more severe anxiety disorders or even depression, trapping individuals in a state of despair where they feel powerless to break free from their cycle of worry.

The impact of chronic worry extends beyond physical and mental health, deeply affecting one's self-confidence and sense of self. As worry takes root, it can erode an individual's confidence in their ability to handle life's challenges. This diminished self-belief can lead to avoidance behaviors, where one may shy away from opportunities or social situations due to fear of failure or embarrassment. Over time, this can reinforce a sense of inadequacy or helplessness, perpetuating a cycle of worry and self-doubt. The individual may start to view the world through a lens of fear and negativity, limiting their potential for growth and fulfillment.

The effects of chronic worry are not confined to the individual; they ripple outward, impacting relationships with loved ones and colleagues. Friends and family members may find it challenging to offer support or empathy to someone perpetually anxious and preoccupied. The constant focus on worst-case scenarios and the inability to be fully present in conversations can strain relationships, leading to feelings of frustration or helplessness in those trying to provide support. Over time, this can create emotional distance, leaving the individual feeling isolated or misunderstood, further fueling their worries and compounding their mental and emotional distress.

Chronic worry in the workplace can significantly hamper productivity and creativity. The inability to concentrate on tasks or make confident decisions can impede performance, decreasing job satisfaction and professional advancement. If one member is consistently anxious, colleagues may observe a lack of engagement or motivation, and managers may notice a decline in overall team morale. Over time, these effects can accumulate, potentially leading to burnout, absenteeism, or even career derailment if not addressed.

Understanding the significant toll of chronic worry is crucial in seeking the proper support and implementing strategies to manage stress. Addressing chronic worry through mindfulness practices, cognitive-behavioral therapy, or lifestyle changes like regular exercise and relaxation techniques can help mitigate its impact. Individuals can reclaim their well-being and build a more balanced, fulfilling life by focusing on what can be controlled and letting go of the rest.

Linda's Journey with Chronic Worry

Linda, a 52-year-old mother of three and a marketing executive, had always been a bit of a worrier. But in her forties, her worry intensified, becoming a constant companion she couldn't shake. She found herself obsessively worrying about her children's futures, her aging parent's declining health, and the stability of her job. Linda's mind would spiral with "what ifs"—What if my son doesn't get into college? What if my parents need full-time care? What if I lose my job? These thoughts would consume her day and often keep her up at night.

Linda's worry reached a tipping point when she began experiencing panic attacks at work. She would become breathless and faint when worrying about her job's instability. Feeling overwhelmed and desperate for relief, she decided to seek help. She started therapy, where she learned to differentiate between productive concern and unproductive worry. Her therapist helped her focus on what she could control, such as creating a financial plan for her children's education and setting up a support network for her parents. Linda was encouraged to practice mindfulness and accept the things she couldn't control.

Gradually, Linda began incorporating mindfulness meditation into her daily routine. She also started keeping a gratitude journal to shift her focus from what could go wrong to what was going right in her life. Over time, Linda felt more at peace and less consumed by worry. She realized that while she couldn't control every aspect of life, she could control how she responded to her thoughts and fears.

Exercise: Recognizing and Challenging Worry Triggers

Set aside a few minutes each day to reflect on your worries. Write them down in a journal, noting the situations or thoughts that triggered each worry. Are these worries based on things you can control, or are they speculative "what if" scenarios? For each worry, ask yourself:

1. Is this worry based on a real or imagined situation?

2. What evidence do I have that this worry will come true?

3. What can I do to address this concern constructively?

4. What can I tell myself to let go of the things I cannot control?

Regularly practicing this exercise will make you more aware of your worry patterns and better equipped to manage them.

Jennifer's Realization About Control

A 45-year-old high school speech therapist, Jennifer had always been a worrier. She was the type who fretted over her students' well-being long after the school bell rang. She would lie awake at night thinking about a student who seemed withdrawn or a teenager whose parents were going through a divorce. Her concern extended far beyond the classroom walls; world events, political instability, and natural disasters often weighed heavily on her mind. She felt a constant undercurrent of anxiety, a nagging unease about things she knew she couldn't control but couldn't stop thinking about either.

Her worries started to take a toll on her health and well-being. Jennifer began to experience tension headaches and difficulty sleeping, her mind racing with endless "what if" scenarios. Her friends and colleagues noticed she seemed distracted and less present in conversations. She knew she needed to change something but wasn't sure what or how. The more she tried to control the external world around her, the more helpless she felt. Her anxiety was becoming an uninvited guest in her life, one that refused to leave no matter how much she tried to reason with it.

The turning point came during a mandatory school workshop on mental health. The speaker, a psychologist specializing in stress management, spoke about the importance of distinguishing between what we can control and what we can't. He introduced a simple yet profound idea: "Control the controllables." Jennifer sat in the back of the room, half-listening, half-preoccupied with her thoughts, when the speaker's words pierced through her cloud of worry. It struck her like a lightning bolt. She realized that much of her anxiety stemmed from trying to control things she had no power over—her students' family issues, global crises, and the unpredictable future.

Inspired, Jennifer decided to put this idea into practice. She started small, focusing on what she could change in her immediate environment. She organized her classroom to be a more calming space, introduced mindfulness exercises at the beginning of her sessions, and set more precise boundaries for her time. Every time she felt the familiar wave of anxiety about something beyond her control—like a news headline or a student's troubled home life—she would gently remind herself: "Control the controllables." This simple mantra became a mental anchor, helping her pull back from the spiral of worry and refocus on what was right in front of her.

Gradually, Jennifer noticed a change. She became more present with her students, engaged in her work, and relaxed in her personal life. Her headaches diminished, and she started sleeping better. She found herself laughing more, enjoying the little moments that once passed her by unnoticed. She began to appreciate the power of letting go—not of caring, but of the need to control everything. Jennifer realized that while she couldn't change the world, she could change how she responded. She learned to find peace in the present, knowing that her energy was better spent on the things within her reach. And in doing so, she discovered a sense of freedom and calm she hadn't felt in years.

Use this space to jot down your thoughts, ideas, and any insights you gain as you work through the book. Let it be a place for reflection, breakthroughs, and practical takeaways that can help guide you toward a more peaceful mind.

_____

_____

_____

_____

_____

_____

_____

_____

_____

_____

_____

_____

_____

_____

_____

_____

_____

_____

Chapter 2

The Science Behind Worry

How Worry Affects the Brain and Body

Chronic worry exacts a significant cost, often creeping into every aspect of life and silently wearing down both the body and mind. Physically, the body responds to prolonged stress by staying alert, usually called the "fight or flight" mode. This constant state of vigilance can lead to various physical symptoms, such as persistent headaches caused by muscle tension in the neck and shoulders or even migraines triggered by stress. The continuous release of stress hormones, such as cortisol, can elevate blood pressure, placing extra strain on the heart and heightening the risk of cardiovascular diseases. Digestive issues, such as acid reflux, irritable bowel syndrome, or stomach ulcers, can also arise from the body's stress response, as chronic worry disrupts normal digestive functions. Also, prolonged stress can weaken the immune system, leaving the body more vulnerable to infections and illnesses and slowing recovery. Mentally, chronic worry can be equally debilitating. The constant barrage of anxious thoughts can lead to overwhelming fatigue as the mind is perpetually engaged in overthinking and scenario-building. This mental exhaustion often spills over into emotional regulation, making individuals more irritable or prone to mood swings. Sleep disturbances, such as insomnia or restless sleep, are common, as worries play on a loop in the mind, preventing restful sleep and leading to a vicious cycle of exhaustion and anxiety. Over time, this relentless mental strain can develop into more severe anxiety disorders or even depression, trapping individuals in a state of despair where they feel powerless to break free from their cycle of worry.

The Worry Loop

The worry loop is a self-perpetuating cycle that begins with an anxious thought, followed by a physiological response (such as a racing heart), leading to more anxious thoughts. This cycle is often fueled by cognitive distortions—irrational thoughts that convince us the worst-case scenario is possible and likely. The longer this loop continues, the more ingrained it becomes, making it harder to break free.

Sarah's Journey into and Out of Worry

Sarah, a 30-year-old woman with bright eyes and a kind heart, had always dreamed of becoming a mother. Her heart swelled with joy and anticipation when she discovered she was pregnant. She imagined all the beautiful moments ahead, feeling her baby kick, decorating the nursery, and holding her little one for the first time. But almost as soon as she felt the joy, a shadow of worry began to creep in. Sarah carried a genetic marker that increased the risk of a specific disability, and there was a 25% chance she could pass it on to her baby. This thought lodged itself deep in her mind, looping endlessly, turning her dreams into a fog of anxiety.

As the weeks passed, Sarah was trapped in a relentless cycle of worry. She would wake up in the middle of the night, heart pounding, convinced something was wrong. Her days were filled with a constant stream of "what ifs." What if her baby was born with a disability? What if she wasn't strong enough to handle it? The fear of the unknown consumed her thoughts. She tried to distract herself by reading baby books and planning for the future, but the worry lurked beneath the surface. The stress began to take a toll on her body. She felt nauseous all the time, unable to eat or sleep properly, and her energy dwindled to a low hum. She started losing weight, and her skin grew pale.

Her husband, Mark, watched helplessly as the woman he loved seemed to wither before his eyes. He tried everything to reassure her—comforting words, warm embraces, and gentle reminders that they were in this together. But no matter what he said, Sarah's fear seemed unshakeable. Her worry was like a heavy fog she couldn't see beyond, a loop that played repeatedly in her mind. Mark was scared, not just for their baby, but for Sarah. He feared she was losing herself to this fear, becoming a shadow of the vibrant woman he knew. He longed to help her find peace, to ease her mind, but he felt powerless against the relentless tide of her anxiety.

One evening, after a challenging day filled with tears and frustration, Sarah realized she couldn't go on like this. She needed to break free from this worry loop that had consumed her life. She decided to face her fear head-on and talk to her doctor about genetic testing. It was a difficult decision; she was terrified of what the test might reveal. But she also knew that living in constant fear was not the answer. With Mark's unwavering support, she went in for the test. The days waiting for the results were some of the hardest of her life, filled with a mix of dread and hope.

When the results finally came in, Sarah held her breath as the doctor spoke. Her baby did not carry the gene. Relief washed over her, and tears streamed down her face. For the first time in months, she felt the heavy weight of worry lift from her shoulders. She realized that her fear, while understandable, had taken over her life and robbed her of the joy of her pregnancy. She hugged Mark tightly, feeling his love and relief envelop her. She knew she could now focus on nurturing the life growing inside her without the constant shadow of fear.

Sarah's journey taught her the power of worry and the importance of confronting her fears with compassion and courage. She learned to be kinder to herself, understanding that her worry was rooted in love and concern, not weakness. But it was making her miss the fun of pregnancy and fun anticipation. With Mark by her side, she moved forward, embracing the rest of her pregnancy with a renewed sense of hope and calm. She knew there would still be challenges ahead, but she also knew she had the strength to face them, one step at a time, with love guiding her.

Worry and Imagination

Worry hijacks our imagination, transforming it from a tool for creativity and problem-solving into a mechanism for anxiety and fear. The same mental faculties that allow us to dream big and visualize positive outcomes are misused to imagine negative scenarios. By becoming aware of this process, we can learn to redirect our imagination toward more constructive, positive uses.

"Our anxiety does not come from thinking about the future, but from wanting to control it."

— Kahlil Gibran

Chapter 3

Mindfulness: The Art of Being Present

Introduction to Mindfulness and Cognitive Restructuring

Mindfulness and cognitive restructuring are two powerful, scientifically supported techniques that can help interrupt the worry loop:

Mindfulness is the practice of focusing on the present moment with an open, accepting, and nonjudgmental mindset. It helps individuals become more aware of their thoughts and feelings without becoming overwhelmed. This awareness can reduce the tendency to ruminate on past mistakes or worry about future fears, which are common components of the worry loop.

Cognitive restructuring involves identifying and challenging irrational thoughts and replacing them with more balanced, rational ones. Cognitive restructuring is a cognitive-behavioral therapy (CBT) technique that focuses on recognizing and challenging irrational or unhelpful thoughts and replacing them with more balanced and rational alternatives. This technique helps individuals recognize patterns of negative thinking that contribute to anxiety and learn to replace them with healthier thought patterns.

Mark's Breakthrough with Cognitive Restructuring

Mark, a 47-year-old entrepreneur, always felt he had to be in control. His business was his life's work, and he worried constantly about its success. "What if the market crashes?" "What if my competitors outmaneuver me?" "What if my best employee leaves?" These 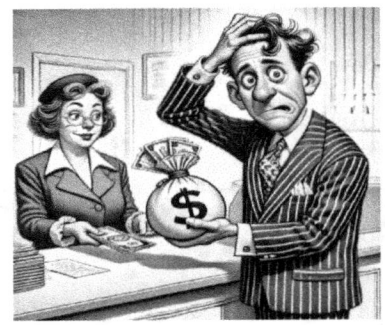 thoughts dominated his mind, leading to chronic migraines, insomnia, and bouts of anxiety.

Mark's breaking point came when his anxiety began affecting his decision-making abilities. Realizing he needed help, he found a Life Coach who introduced him to cognitive restructuring techniques. With her guidance, Mark started journaling his worries, documenting the evidence for and against each worry, and reframing them with more balanced positive thoughts.

For example, instead of thinking, "If the market crashes, my business will fail," Mark reframed, "While a market crash could pose challenges, I have a solid business model and a loyal customer base. I can adapt and find new strategies if needed." Over time, this practice helped Mark break free from the cycle of catastrophic thinking. He felt more empowered and confident in his ability to handle challenges, transforming his relationship with his business and mind.

"Do not anticipate trouble or worry about what may never happen. Keep in the sunlight."

— Benjamin Franklin

Exercise: Cognitive Restructuring Practice

Keep a "Thought Record" to track your worries and practice cognitive restructuring. For each worry, write down:

1. The Situation: What triggered the worry?

2. The Automatic Thought: What was the initial worry or negative thought?

3. The Emotion: What feelings did this thought evoke?

4. Evidence for the Thought: Does any evidence support this worry?

5. Evidence Against the Thought: What evidence exists that contradicts the worry?

6. Alternative Thought: Write a balanced thought that acknowledges both sides and reframes the situation more positively.

Reflect on how this exercise helps shift your mindset from fear to rational thinking. Review your journal weekly to track progress and identify patterns or recurring themes.

Dana's Journey of Self-Awareness

Dana, a 45-year-old single mom and software developer, had always been prone to overthinking. Her days were filled with constant worries—about her job security, her children's education, the state of the economy, and the endless tasks of daily life. Adding to her stress, Dana's elderly mother had recently moved in with her, needing more support as her health declined. Caring for her mom was emotionally and physically exhausting, especially with the added challenge of her aging dog, who sometimes peed in the house, adding another layer of frustration to her already full plate. Her home, once a sanctuary, now felt like a pressure cooker, with one thing after another vying for her attention and mental energy.

Dana's worries often spiraled out of control, keeping her awake at night, replaying worst-case scenarios. She noticed herself becoming increasingly irritable, snapping at her kids over minor issues, and feeling disconnected from them and her mom. Her anxiety seemed to seep into every corner of her life, making it hard to focus on her work as a software developer, where job security always felt like it hung in the balance. She constantly checked her emails, fearing bad news, and her mind was always racing with thoughts of what could go wrong next.

Things began to change after Dana attended a workshop on cognitive restructuring. For the first time, she learned about cognitive distortions—the irrational, exaggerated thought patterns that were driving her anxiety. She realized she had been caught in a cycle of catastrophizing, jumping to conclusions, and seeing everything in black-and-white terms. This newfound awareness was like a light bulb going off. She systematically challenged these distorted thoughts, questioning their validity and considering more balanced, realistic perspectives.

As Dana practiced this new approach, she noticed a significant reduction in her anxiety levels. She began to feel more in control of her thoughts and less overwhelmed by them. Her newfound self-awareness had a ripple effect on her entire life. She became less irritable and more present with her family, able to enjoy moments with her kids without the constant cloud of worry hanging over her. She found new patience in caring for her mother, understanding that she and her mom were doing their best in a difficult situation. Even the mishaps with her elderly dog became more manageable, no longer feeling like the end of the world.

Dana's journey towards managing her worry was transformative. She learned that while she couldn't control every aspect of her life, she could control how she responded to her thoughts. This shift improved her mental well-being and strengthened her relationships with her family. She 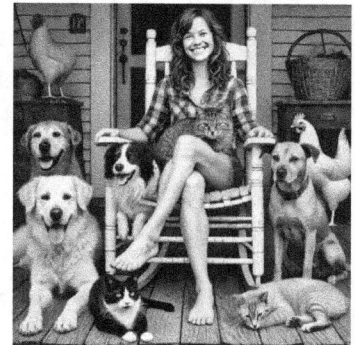 felt more connected, compassionate, and capable of handling life's ups and downs with a calm, steady heart.

Understanding Mindfulness

Mindfulness is being fully present in the moment, aware of your thoughts, feelings, and sensations without judgment. It is a skill that helps interrupt the worry cycle by grounding you in the present rather than allowing your mind to drift into anxious thoughts about the future. Mindfulness has roots in ancient meditation traditions but has gained popularity in modern psychology as a powerful tool for reducing stress and anxiety.

Techniques for Practicing Mindfulness

1. **Breathing Exercises:** Focused breathing helps calm the nervous system. Practice "4-7-8 breathing": inhale through your nose for four counts, hold for seven counts, and exhale through your mouth for eight counts. This technique

promotes relaxation and can be done anywhere, anytime you feel worried or stressed.

2. **Body Scans:** A body scan meditation involves mentally looking at your body from head to toe and noticing any sensations or areas of tension. This practice fosters a deeper connection with your body, eases stress, and encourages relaxation. You can perform it while lying down, sitting, or even standing.

3. **Mindful Walking:** Practice walking meditation by focusing on the sensations of your feet touching the ground, the rhythm of your steps, and the sounds surrounding you. Redirecting your attention from your thoughts to your physical experience keeps you anchored in the present moment, helping to alleviate worry.

4. **Mindful Eating:** When you eat, focus entirely on the experience—the taste, texture, and aroma of your food. Eating mindfully can enhance your appreciation for the present moment and reduce stress-related eating habits.

Exercise: 30-Day Mindfulness Challenge

Commit to a 30-day mindfulness challenge, during which you will practice mindfulness for at least 10 minutes daily. Rotate through different mindfulness techniques to find what works best for you. Keep a journal of your experiences, noting any changes in your worry patterns, mood, and overall well-being. Consider setting a specific time each day for your practice, such as first thing in the morning or right before bed, to help establish a consistent routine.

Susan's Transformation Through Mindfulness

Susan, a 45-year-old nurse, was no stranger to high-pressure situations. She had spent years caring for her patients with unwavering dedication, often working long hours and dealing with life-and-death scenarios. But lately, her worries had started to pile up, weighing heavily on her heart. She worried about her patients—wondering if she had done enough, if they would recover, or if she could have done something differently. But her worries didn't end when she left the hospital. They followed her home, seeping into every corner of her life, disrupting her sleep, and leaving her with a deep sense of chronic fatigue.

Susan's concerns extended beyond her professional life. She was deeply worried about her sister, Sandy, who struggled with addiction and had been out of touch for months. Every time the phone rang, Susan's heart would skip a beat, hoping Sandy was reaching out, yet dreading bad news. She felt a constant ache in her chest, a mixture of fear and helplessness, as she imagined the worst-case scenarios. Susan also couldn't shake the worry about the young boy across the street. She had seen him sneaking out at night, his small frame darting through the shadows, and she feared for his safety, wondering if he was okay or if he had someone looking out for him.

Her worries began to consume her. She was constantly on edge, her mind racing from one fear to another. Her sleep was restless, filled with anxious dreams, and she woke up each morning more exhausted than the last. Her fatigue became a constant companion, making her feel as though she was moving through life with a heavy weight on her shoulders. She knew she needed to find a way to break free from this cycle of worry, but she didn't know how.

After a particularly challenging week, Susan decided to attend a mindfulness workshop at a friend's suggestion. She was skeptical—mindfulness seemed a bit too woo-woo for her practical, no-nonsense approach to life. But she was also intrigued by the idea of finding some peace of mind amidst the chaos. At the workshop, she learned simple techniques like mindful breathing and mindful walking, practices that invited her to focus on the present moment instead of getting lost in anxious thoughts.

She began incorporating these practices into her daily routine, starting with a few minutes of mindful breathing each morning and a mindful walk during her lunch breaks. The effects were gradual, but over time, Susan noticed a shift. She found herself worrying less and becoming more present in her daily activities. She started to feel more attuned to her needs, recognizing when to rest, ask for help, and breathe through a difficult moment. Her newfound mindfulness practice taught her to be more compassionate toward herself, acknowledging her worries without letting them take over. She also became more empathetic toward others, offering kindness to her patients, her family, and herself.

Susan's mindfulness practice became a vital part of her routine, a daily refuge that helped her navigate her stresses more calmly and clearly. She learned that while she couldn't control everything in her life—her patients' outcomes, her sister's choices, or the young boy's situation—she could control how she responded to her thoughts and emotions. This realization brought a profound sense of peace, allowing her to approach each day with a more open heart and a gentler spirit, grounded in the present moment and the love that connected her to those she cared about.

"Worry often gives a small thing a big shadow."

— Swedish Proverb

Rachel's Mindfulness Journey with Family Dynamics

Rachel, a 39-year-old single mother, often found herself lying awake at night, worried about her teenage daughter, Lily. Lately,

Lily had been spending too much time with a crowd Rachel wasn't sure about, and her constant attachment to her phone deepened Rachel's concerns. She feared Lily was drifting away, caught up in influences and distractions that could lead her down the wrong path.

Rachel's anxiety spiked every time Lily stayed out late or seemed glued to her screen, her face illuminated by a world Rachel couldn't see or understand. She felt powerless, afraid that Lily might make choices with long-term consequences that Rachel couldn't control or protect her from. The more Rachel tried to intervene, the more she felt their bond fraying, with arguments becoming frequent and their once warm conversations turning cold and tense.

Desperate for a change, Rachel stumbled upon mindfulness on a website and decided to try it. At first, it seemed too simple—just being present and listening without judgment. But as she began to practice mindful communication, she noticed a shift. Instead of jumping to conclusions or reacting with frustration when Lily's phone buzzed late at night, Rachel would take a deep breath and focus on listening. She approached conversations with curiosity rather than criticism, asking open-ended questions and genuinely wanting to understand her daughter's perspective.

To her surprise, this new approach began to work. Lily started to open up more, sharing her thoughts and feelings about her friends and the pressures she faced. She felt more understood and less judged, and in turn, she began to spend less time on her phone and more time engaging in their conversations. Rachel realized her daughter wasn't lost in a digital world or succumbing to bad influences; she was navigating the complex terrain of teenage life, just like any other teenager.

Through mindfulness, Rachel found a way to transform her worries into opportunities for connection. It helped her see that fostering trust and understanding was more powerful than trying to control every aspect of her daughter's life. As their relationship deepened, Rachel's anxiety faded, replaced by a newfound confidence in Lily's ability to make her own choices—knowing she had a strong foundation of love and support to guide her.

Use this space to jot down your thoughts, ideas, and any insights you gain as you work through the book. Let it be a place for reflection, breakthroughs, and practical takeaways that can help guide you toward a more peaceful mind.

_____

_____

_____

_____

_____

_____

_____

_____

_____

_____

_____

_____

_____

_____

_____

_____

_____

_____

Chapter 4

Cognitive Behavioral Techniques to Reduce Worry

Introduction to Cognitive Behavioral Therapy (CBT)

Cognitive Behavioral Therapy (CBT) is a powerful method for managing worry and anxiety. It is rooted in the concept that our thoughts, feelings, and behaviors are closely linked. By changing our thoughts, we can change our emotions and behaviors. CBT provides a framework for identifying and challenging negative thought patterns, helping us develop healthier, more balanced ways of thinking.

Techniques for Identifying and Challenging Negative Thoughts

1. **Thought Records:** Use thought records to track worried thoughts and identify patterns. For each worry, write down the situation, the negative thought, the associated emotion, and evidence for and against the thought. This practice helps you see your worries more objectively.

2. **Cognitive Restructuring:** Identify cognitive distortions such as catastrophizing (assuming the worst will happen), overgeneralization (believing that one adverse event is part of a pattern), and all-or-nothing thinking (seeing things in black-and-white terms). Practice reframing these thoughts into more balanced, rational perspectives.

3. **The "ABCDE" Model:** The ABCDE model (Adversity, Belief, Consequence, Disputation, Energization) provides a structured approach to challenging irrational thoughts and replacing them with more constructive ones.

Exercise: Cognitive Behavioral Techniques Practice

Create a "Worry Journal" where you document your worries using the ABCDE model:

- **Adversity:** Describe the situation that triggered your worry.

- **Belief:** Identify the worry or negative thought.

- **Consequence:** Note the emotional and behavioral response to the belief.

- **Disputation:** Challenge the belief by asking, "Is this thought true? What evidence do I have against it?"

- **Energization:** Create a new, more balanced belief and note how this new belief makes you feel.

Review your journal weekly to track progress and identify patterns or recurring themes. This exercise helps you develop a habit of questioning and reframing worried thoughts.

Carol's Success with Thought Records

Carol, a 48-year-old high school teacher, was a master at maintaining order in her classroom, but outside those four walls, she often felt like her life was spinning out of control. Her days were filled with a constant stream of worries. She would find herself fretting over her students' futures—wondering if she had done enough to prepare them for the world beyond school. Then, there was her career stability, an ever-present concern in a world where educational funding and policies seemed to shift like quicksand. And as if that wasn't enough, Carol also cared for her aging parents, who required increasing time and energy.

These worries had a way of compounding, spiraling into an endless loop of anxious thoughts that left Carol feeling overwhelmed and exhausted. She often lay awake at night, her mind racing from one worry to the next, unable to shut off the cascade of what-ifs and worst-case scenarios. It felt like every aspect of her life was a potential minefield, ready to explode at any moment. The stress was taking a toll on her health, relationships, and overall well-being.

One day, during a rare coffee break with a close friend, Carol confided in her about the constant anxiety that seemed to grip her life. Her friend listened attentively and then suggested she try using thought records, a cognitive-behavioral technique designed to manage stress by examining and restructuring one's thoughts. Carol was skeptical. She had always been the type to handle things independently, and the idea of writing down her worries felt a bit... gimmicky. But she was also desperate for relief, so she tried it.

Armed with a notebook, Carol began documenting her worries each day. She followed the ABCDE model: **A**ctivating event, **B**elief, **C**onsequences, **D**ispute, and **E**ffect. At first, it was challenging to confront her thoughts head-on. She had always just accepted them as part of who she was—a worrier by nature. But as she dissected each worry, she began to see patterns. Many of her anxieties were based on irrational fears or assumptions. For instance, her worry that her students would fail in life wasn't based on concrete evidence; it was rooted in her fear of not being good enough as a teacher. Similarly, her dread over her job security was often triggered by vague rumors or her interpretation of a colleague's offhand comment rather than factual information.

With this newfound clarity, Carol began challenging her thoughts. She asked herself tough questions: "Is there any real evidence to support this worry?" or "Am I catastrophizing?" She started replacing those automatic negative thoughts with more balanced, realistic perspectives. Instead of thinking, "I'm a failure if one of my students doesn't succeed," she would remind herself, "I'm doing my best to equip my students with the tools they need; their success also depends on their efforts and choices."

Gradually, Carol noticed a shift. The grip of her worries loosened, and she no longer felt as paralyzed by anxiety. However, records had become a powerful tool for her, managing her immediate worries and fostering a deeper understanding of herself and her triggers. The process gave her the space to pause, reflect, and choose how to respond rather than reacting impulsively out of fear.

As weeks turned into months, Carol's confidence grew. She began to feel more in control, not just in her classroom but in her life. Her success with thought records also sparked a ripple effect—her relationships with her parents improved as she became more present and less preoccupied with anxiety. She even found herself more engaged with her students, encouraging them to explore mindfulness and self-awareness techniques she had learned.

Carol's journey with thought records wasn't a magic fix, but it was a transformative step towards reclaiming her life from the clutches of chronic worry. She had learned that while she couldn't control every outcome or predict the future, she could control her responses to her thoughts. And that realization brought a sense of peace and resilience she hadn't felt in years. With her notebook and new mindset, Carol was ready to face challenges, knowing she had the tools to navigate them with grace and confidence.

"The greatest mistake you can make in life is to continually fear you will make one."

— Elbert Hubbard

Nathan's Use of Cognitive Techniques in Leadership

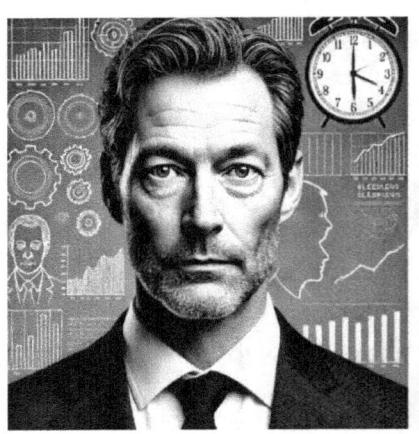

Nathan, a 52-year-old corporate executive, was no stranger to pressure. He appeared confident and composed on the outside, the leader who could easily command a room. But behind closed doors, Nathan's mind was a storm of self-doubt and worry. He often lay awake at night, staring at the ceiling, replaying the day's decisions repeatedly, second-guessing every choice he had made. "Was that strategy too risky?" "Did I handle that meeting well enough?" "What if the company's future is jeopardized because of me?"

Nathan's worries were relentless, gnawing away at him. He felt the weight of his responsibilities not just as a leader but as a protector of the livelihoods of hundreds of employees. Every decision seemed to carry the potential for catastrophe in his mind. A fear of failure constantly plagued him—a fear that he wasn't truly capable of steering the company in the right direction. This anxiety often spilled over into his personal life, where he struggled to be present with his family, his thoughts constantly drifting back to work to what could go wrong next.

One day, after a particularly stressful board meeting, Nathan's closest friend and colleague noticed his exhaustion and suggested he investigate Cognitive Behavioral Therapy (CBT). Nathan was skeptical. Therapy had always seemed like something for people who couldn't handle stress, and he had always prided himself on his resilience. But he was tired of feeling on edge, tired of the sleepless nights. He only explored CBT to see if it might offer some relief.

He learned about thought records, a technique for tracking and analyzing negative thoughts. Initially, the process felt awkward and forced. Writing down his worries seemed like an admission of weakness, and it was challenging for someone who had spent years cultivating a tough exterior. But as he started documenting his anxious thoughts, something surprising happened: Nathan began recognizing patterns. His fears often stemmed from catastrophizing—imagining the worst possible outcomes—and from an all-or-nothing mindset, where every decision was seen as either a complete success or a devastating failure.

Using the CBT framework, Nathan began to challenge these thoughts. When he thought, "If this project fails, the whole company could go under," he would stop and ask, "Is this true? What evidence do I have? What's the worst that could realistically happen?" He started to see that many of his worries were based more on emotion than fact. He began reframing his thoughts: instead of seeing decisions as potential disasters, he started to view them as experiments—opportunities to learn and grow, even if things didn't go perfectly.

This shift in mindset didn't happen overnight, but gradually, Nathan began to feel a change. The constant knot of anxiety in his chest began to loosen. He found himself sleeping better, waking up feeling more rested and clear-headed. In meetings, he was more present, more open to collaboration and feedback, and less paralyzed by the fear of making mistakes. His newfound perspective not only made him a more confident leader but also a more empathetic one. He began to share his challenges with his team, creating an environment where mistakes were seen not as failures but as stepping stones to success.

Nathan's journey with CBT and thought records transformed more than just his professional life. It allowed him to reconnect with his family, to be more present at the dinner table, and to engage more fully in his children's lives. He realized that his worth as a leader and person wasn't defined by avoiding failure but by his ability to learn, adapt, and grow from every experience. This shift brought a profound sense of peace, realizing he didn't have to be perfect to be effective. He just had to be willing to face his fears, challenge his thoughts, and embrace the journey with a sense of curiosity and openness.

With this new mindset, Nathan became a better leader and a more fulfilled person, ready to face the complexities of his role with courage and resilience. He learned that true strength lay not in being unshakable but in being willing to be vulnerable, learn, and grow. In this, he found a new kind of confidence grounded not in fear but in the freedom to lead with authenticity and heart.

Use this space to jot down your thoughts, ideas, and any insights you gain as you work through the book. Let it be a place for reflection, breakthroughs, and practical takeaways that can help guide you toward a more peaceful mind.

_____

_____

_____

_____

_____

_____

_____

_____

_____

_____

_____

_____

_____

_____

_____

_____

_____

_____

Chapter 5

The Power of Imagination: Reclaiming Your Creative Mind

Imagination vs. Worry

Imagination is a powerful tool that fuels worry, creativity, and problem-solving. When we worry, we use our imagination to envision negative outcomes and catastrophes. However, by learning to redirect this mental energy, we can harness imagination to create positive, constructive visions for the future.

Techniques to Reclaim Imagination for Positive Use

1. **Creative Visualization:** This technique involves vividly imagining a positive outcome. Picture yourself successfully navigating a challenging situation, focusing on this favorable scenario's sights, sounds, and feelings.

2. **Daydreaming for Stress Relief:** Allow yourself to daydream without restriction. Imagine ideal situations or scenarios that bring you joy or peace. This practice helps shift your focus from worry to positive, creative thinking.

3. **Using Imagination to Solve Problems:** Instead of focusing on potential problems, use your imagination to brainstorm creative solutions. Visualize yourself overcoming obstacles and achieving your goals.

Exercise: Guided Visualization

Practice a guided visualization exercise for 10 minutes daily. Sit comfortably, breathe deeply, close your eyes, and imagine a situation that worries you. Then, visualize a positive outcome, focusing on how you would feel, who would be involved, and what steps you would take. Write down these visualizations in a journal and reflect on any changes in your worry levels or mindset.

John's Journey from Worry to Imagination

John, a 50-year-old engineer, had always seen the world through the lens of practicality and logic. He was the guy who calculated the most efficient way to stack groceries in the car and could predict the lifespan of a light bulb with unsettling accuracy. His family lovingly called him "Safety Sam," a nickname that always made him roll his eyes, but secretly, he took pride in it. After all, what was wrong with being cautious and prepared?

However, John's love for planning and predicting potential problems often spiraled into excessive worrying. Whether it was a leaky faucet at home or a minor hiccup in a project at work, John could turn it into a full-blown disaster scenario faster than you could say "probability." So, when his daughter, Emily, announced her grand plan to take a gap year and travel abroad, John's mind went into a tailspin.

He pictured every possible catastrophe: lost passports, sketchy hostels, strange foreign diseases that he'd have to Google late at night, and don't even get him started on the whole "hitchhiking" idea she casually mentioned. He imagined her backpacking through jungles with giant mosquitoes, getting lost in remote villages with no Wi-Fi, and somehow ending up in a local prison because she didn't understand the customs.

One afternoon, after John had spent an hour on a YouTube deep dive about the dangers of foreign tap water, his good friend Larry decided it was time for an intervention. "John, buddy," Larry said, chuckling, "You need to lighten up. Have you ever thought about trying creative visualization?"

John squinted at him. "Creative what-now?"

"Visualization," Larry repeated. "Instead of focusing on everything that could go wrong, why not imagine everything going right? Picture Emily having the time of her life, making friends, learning new things…you know, thriving."

John raised an eyebrow. "You mean, like, daydream? I'm an engineer, Larry. I deal in facts and figures, not…fantasies."

But that night, lying in bed, John stared at the ceiling, unable to shake Larry's suggestion. He figured he had nothing to lose. So, he decided to give this "visualization" thing a try, albeit reluctantly.

At first, it felt ridiculous. He closed his eyes and tried to conjure up a scene where Emily confidently navigated a bustling market, chatting with locals and bargaining like a pro. But then, his imagination took a turn. Instead of picturing disaster, he saw her leading a spontaneous dance party in the town square, teaching everyone the "Electric Slide." He saw her standing atop a mountain, arms spread wide, with a grin that said, "I've conquered this!"

Surprisingly, the more he practiced, the more vivid and joyful these visualizations became. He saw Emily meeting a quirky group of international friends, bonding over strange foods, and laughing until their sides hurt. He even started imagining silly scenarios: Emily accidentally joining a parade because she thought it was a walking tour or mistaking a statue for a real person and striking up a conversation. The absurdity made him chuckle, and slowly but surely, his worries began to fade.

John's newfound hobby didn't just stop there. He found himself using visualization techniques at work, too. During a particularly tricky engineering problem, instead of fixating on all the ways a project could fail, he imagined himself as an engineering superhero, cape and all, swooping in with creative solutions. He pictured the parts of his projects not just fitting together but doing so with a triumphant "ta-da!" and a round of applause from his coworkers. The meetings in his head started ending with spontaneous confetti showers, courtesy of his overactive imagination.

As weeks passed, John's entire outlook began to change. He was no longer the guy who worried excessively about the slightest hiccup. Instead, he approached challenges with a light-hearted sense of humor and optimism. At family dinners, he shared stories about his "adventures in visualization," much to the amusement of Emily and his wife, who both delighted in his newfound whimsical side.

John's journey from worry to imagination transformed his life. He realized that life didn't always need to be approached with caution and fear; sometimes, it could be tackled with creativity and a good laugh. His daughter's upcoming adventure no longer felt like a looming threat but an exciting chapter he could share, even if just in his mind's eye. And as for his engineering work? Well, it seemed a little more fun when you imagined solving problems with a side of confetti.

"Be kind to yourself. You're doing the best you can under the circumstances."

— Joanne Harvey

Anna's Creative Transformation

A 43-year-old marketing manager, Anna was the queen of creativity at work. Known for her out-of-the-box campaigns and brilliant brainstorming sessions, she could turn the most mundane product into something people couldn't wait to buy. But at home, her imagination often ran wild in a different, less fun direction—straight into the depths of worry, especially when it came to her teenage son, Max.

Max was a bright kid, but like most teens, he wasn't thrilled about spending his free time buried in textbooks. His grades were average, and his motivation for schoolwork hovered somewhere between "meh" and "can't be bothered." Anna's mind, ever the imaginative machine, spun into overdrive. She pictured him living in her basement at age 30, surrounded by half-empty pizza boxes, still trying to "find himself." She saw a future filled with missed opportunities and wasted potential, all because he hadn't "applied himself" in high school.

One particularly sleepless night, after envisioning Max as a 40-year-old man-child starting a failed mime troupe in a desperate attempt to make something of his life, Anna decided enough was enough. "I've got to get a grip," she thought. "I use my creativity every day at work to solve problems. Why not use it here?"

With that, Anna hatched a plan to reclaim her imagination from worry and put it to better use. She started with visualization exercises but wasn't content with the basics. Oh no, she turned it into a full-blown production. She imagined Max as the star of a blockbuster movie called "Max's Amazing Life," complete with a rousing soundtrack and a montage of him nailing his goals. There he was, graduating at the top of his class, starting a tech company, giving TED Talks, and even rescuing a kitten from a burning building—all with a confident grin.

But Anna didn't stop there. She grabbed a bunch of magazines, scissors, and glue and created a vision board that could rival any modern art masterpiece. It was filled with images of inspiring leaders, dream colleges, exciting career paths, and motivational quotes like "Believe in yourself!" and "Dream Big!" She even threw in a few pictures of kittens, just in case Max needed a reminder that good deeds go a long way.

As she pieced together the vision board, a funny thing happened. Anna felt her anxiety starting to melt away. Instead of dreading Max's future, she began to feel hopeful and energized. She realized she could use her creative talents to visualize success and brainstorm ways to help Max find his path.

Anna decided to get a little more hands-on. She thought about Max's interests—gaming, building things, and, strangely enough, cooking. She saw an opportunity. Why not make these interests the focal point of his studies? She challenged Max to create a video game for his history project, turning the French Revolution into an epic battle royale. For science, she encouraged him to build a working volcano model that could double as a hot sauce dispenser—a guaranteed A+ for ingenuity!

She also introduced "mini victory" celebrations. When Max finished a book, they'd have a mini party with cupcakes and a small gift (often related to his next assignment). When he aced a test, she'd blast his favorite song, and they'd dance around the living room like nobody was watching. The victories were small, but the impact was huge. Seeing his mother's excitement and support, Max began to feel more motivated. He started setting goals inspired by the quirky, creative ways his mom celebrated his efforts.

As the months passed, Anna noticed a remarkable change. Her son was more engaged in his studies, his grades improved, and most importantly, he seemed happier. Anna, too, felt a shift. She was no longer stuck in a cycle of worry; she was enjoying watching her son discover his potential.

One day, Max came home grinning and announced he'd joined the robotics club. "It's actually pretty cool, Mom," he said, showing her a robot he'd helped build that could fetch snacks (his favorite feature). Anna couldn't help but laugh. Here was her son, thriving in ways she hadn't even imagined.

By turning her creative energy from worry into action, Anna helped her son discover his interests and strengths and found a way to reconnect with him in a fun and meaningful way. She realized that reclaiming her imagination wasn't just about managing her anxiety but about using it to inspire and motivate the people she loved most.

Anna's story is a testament to the power of creativity. It shows that we can turn our worries into wonders with some imagination and heart, crafting a bright, bold future full of unexpected joys.

"You can't pour from an empty cup. Take care of yourself first."

— Unknown

Use this space to jot down your thoughts, ideas, and any insights you gain as you work through the book. Let it be a place for reflection, breakthroughs, and practical takeaways that can help guide you toward a more peaceful mind.

_____

_____

_____

_____

_____

_____

_____

_____

_____

_____

_____

_____

_____

_____

_____

_____

_____

_____

Chapter 6

Building Emotional Resilience

Understanding Emotional Resilience

Emotional resilience is the ability to adapt and bounce back from stress, adversity, and setbacks. It's not about avoiding difficulties but learning to face them with strength and grace. Building emotional resilience is crucial for managing worry because it helps us feel more equipped to handle life's challenges.

Techniques for Building Resilience

1. **Positive Self-Talk:** Replace negative self-talk with positive affirmations. Instead of saying, "I can't handle this," try saying, "I have the strength and resources to overcome any challenge."

2. **Developing a Growth Mindset:** Embrace that setbacks are growth opportunities. Recognize that every challenge is a chance to learn and develop new skills.

3. **Practicing Gratitude:** Focus on the positive aspects of your life by practicing gratitude. This mindset shift

helps reduce worry by reminding you of the good things in your life.

4. **Strengthening Emotional Regulation Skills:** Learn techniques to manage intense emotions, such as deep breathing, grounding exercises, and relaxation techniques. These skills help you stay calm and focused when faced with stress.

Exercise: Building a Resilience Toolkit: Steps and Process

Creating a "Resilience Toolkit" is a proactive way to manage worry and build emotional strength. This toolkit is a collection of strategies, practices, and activities that help you stay grounded, relaxed, and positive when anxiety or stress arises. Here's how to build your own Resilience Toolkit:

Step 1: Identify Your Needs and Triggers

Reflect on Your Worry Patterns: Take some time to think about what triggers your worry. Are they specific situations, like work stress or family issues? Or is it general anxiety about the future? Understanding what causes your worry can help you choose the most effective tools for your toolkit.

Consider Your Emotional and Physical Needs: When you feel anxious, consider what you need. Do you need to calm your mind, relax your body, or both? Identifying these needs will guide you in selecting the right techniques.

Step 2: Gather Your Tools

1. Positive Affirmations:

Write down a list of affirmations that resonate with you. These are positive statements that help challenge and overcome self-sabotaging and negative thoughts. Examples include:

- "I am capable and strong."
- "I have the power to choose how I respond to challenges."
- "I am enough just as I am."
- "I am smart and fun to be with."

Keep these affirmations in a notebook or on your phone, where you can easily access them when needed.

2. Grounding Techniques:

Choose grounding techniques that help anchor you in the present moment, such as:

5-4-3-2-1 Technique: Identify five things you can see, four things you can touch, three things you can hear, two things you can smell, and one thing you can taste.

Breathing Exercises: To calm your nervous system, practice deep, slow breathing. Try the 4-7-8 technique: inhale for 4 seconds, hold for 7 seconds, and exhale for 8 seconds.

Practice these techniques regularly so they become second nature when you need them most.

3. Relaxation Exercises:

Incorporate relaxation exercises that help release physical tension and promote calmness, such as:

Progressive Muscle Relaxation: Tense and then release different muscle groups in your body, starting from your toes and moving up to your head.

Guided Imagery: Listen to recordings or visualize calming scenes, like a peaceful beach or a serene forest.

You can include links or resources to guided meditations or relaxation audio tracks.

4. Activities that Bring Joy and Comfort:

List activities that bring you joy, comfort, and peace. These could be hobbies, physical activities, or creative outlets like:

Journaling: Writing down your thoughts and feelings can help you process emotions and gain perspective.

Walking in Nature: Spending time outdoors can help reduce stress and improve mood.

Listening to Music or Podcasts: Choose uplifting music or inspiring podcasts that help shift your focus from worry to positivity.

Create a list of go-to activities you can engage in when feeling overwhelmed.

Step 3: Organize Your Toolkit

Keep It Accessible: Store your Resilience Toolkit in a place where you can easily access it, whether it's a physical notebook, a folder on your computer, or an app on your phone. Make sure it's organized so you can quickly find the right tool.

Create a "Quick Reference" Guide: Include a one-page summary of your most effective techniques so you can quickly refer to them in moments of stress.

Step 4: Practice Regularly

Incorporate Tools into Your Daily Routine: Make using your toolkit a regular habit, not just something you reach for in a crisis. This could mean starting your day with affirmations, taking a few minutes for mindful breathing during lunch, or ending the day with a relaxation exercise.

Set Reminders: Use reminders on your phone or calendar to practice these techniques regularly and ensure they become ingrained in your daily routine.

Step 5: Evaluate and Update Your Toolkit

- Reflect on Effectiveness: Periodically assess which tools work best for you and which are less effective. Reflect on how you feel after using each technique and whether it helps alleviate your worry.

Add New Tools: Stay open to discovering new techniques. Attend workshops, read books, or talk to others about what works for them. Add any new tools that resonate with you.

Remove or Adapt Less Effective Tools: If specific techniques are not working as well as expected, consider adapting them or removing them from your toolkit.

Step 6: Share and Expand Your Toolkit

Share with Loved Ones: Sharing your Resilience Toolkit with family or friends can help create a supportive environment and encourage others to build their resilience.

Expand for Different Situations: Create variations of your toolkit tailored for specific situations, such as work stress, family conflicts, or personal anxieties. This way, you'll have targeted strategies ready for different scenarios.

By building a personalized Resilience Toolkit, you empower yourself with a range of strategies to manage worry effectively. Regular practice and thoughtful updates to your toolkit can help you stay resilient, grounded, and prepared 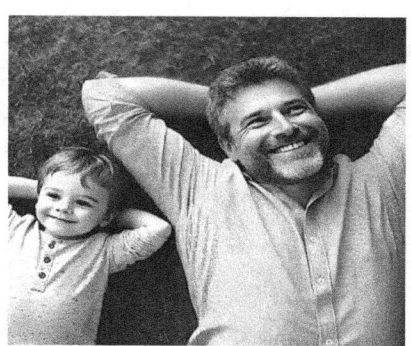 to face life's challenges with greater peace and confidence.

Emma's Path to Resilience

Emma, a 62-year-old accountant, was not just any accountant— she was a powerhouse in her field. Emma was known for her precision, dedication, and unwavering work ethic and was her firm's go-to person for complex financial audits and strategic planning. She had a reputation for turning chaos into order, balancing the books with such finesse that her colleagues joked she could make the numbers dance. She was respected and admired professionally, but beneath her poised exterior, Emma was a chronic worrier. Her worries ran deep and wide, touching every corner of her life. She constantly fretted about making a mistake at

49

work despite her stellar record. She worried about her teenage son, Liam, who was going through a rebellious phase and seemed disinterested in his future. She feared for her aging parents' health, feeling the weight of their care on her shoulders. Even her aging dog's increasingly frequent accidents in the house added to her stress. Emma's mind was a revolving door of what-ifs and worst-case scenarios, and these relentless thoughts often kept her awake at night. As a result, she spent her days feeling tired, irritable, and on edge—a stark contrast to the calm, collected professional everyone saw.

The turning point came when Emma attended a workshop on emotional resilience, somewhat reluctantly, after a persistent friend urged her to go. She walked into the room skeptically, convinced that no positive thinking could shift her deeply ingrained worries. But as the workshop progressed, something in her began to soften. The facilitator discussed building a "Resilience Toolkit" with practical strategies to manage worry and stress. They explained that this toolkit could include techniques like positive self-talk, grounding exercises, and activities that bring joy and comfort. These concepts, which Emma had always dismissed as too "touchy-feely" for her pragmatic mindset, suddenly seemed more accessible. Maybe it was the way the facilitator spoke or the heartfelt stories shared by other attendees about their transformations. Or perhaps it was the sheer exhaustion from years of carrying the world's weight on her shoulders. Whatever it was, Emma decided to give it a try. She figured she had nothing to lose and a lot to gain.

Emma started by incorporating positive self-talk into her daily routine as the first tool in her Resilience Toolkit. At first, it felt awkward, almost contrived, to stand in front of the mirror and tell herself she was strong, capable, and enough. But she persisted. She wrote down affirmations like, "I am resilient," "I am doing my best," and "I am capable of handling whatever comes my way." She taped them to her bathroom mirror, her computer monitor at work, and even the dashboard of her car. Slowly, these words became less like lies and more like possibilities. She added grounding techniques, such as mindful breathing and sensory awareness, to her toolkit to complement this whenever she felt overwhelmed by worry—whether about a looming deadline at work, Liam's behavior, or her parent's health—she would take a few deep breaths and focus on the present moment, using the 5-4-3-2-1 technique to ground herself in reality.

Emma also introduced activities that brought her joy and comfort into her toolkit. She began keeping a gratitude journal on her bedside table, challenging herself to write down five things she was grateful for each night. At first, it was a struggle—her mind, so accustomed to focusing on problems and potential pitfalls, balked at the idea of finding joy in the mundane. She used the five senses. taste, sound, scent, touch, and sight. She stated that it was small: the taste was warm from a cup of tea in the morning, the sound of a bird singing, the smell of cranberries, the happy touch of her dog, and the sunshine on her way to work. She always challenged herself to find something new. As days turned into weeks, Emma noticed a shift. Her list of gratitude grew longer and more varied. She began to see beauty in the little things she had previously overlooked: the laughter of a child, the feel of rain on her face, the satisfaction of a job well done.

As Emma continued to build and use her Resilience Toolkit, she noticed a significant change in her perspective and well-being. She felt lighter and more capable of handling life's challenges. When her teenager, Liam, came home with a poor report card, she approached him with empathy and a willingness to understand his struggles instead of spiraling into worry about his future. She found creative ways to engage with him, tapping into her newfound resilience to help him discover his path. She began to see her parents' aging not as a looming crisis but as an opportunity to connect more deeply, cherishing every moment with them. Even her dog's accidents became less of a frustration and more of a reminder of the importance of patience, taking him on more walks, and love he's sweet temperament.

At work, her newfound emotional resilience shone through. Emma became not just a problem-solver but a beacon of positivity. Her colleagues noticed her transformation; she was still the same sharp, meticulous accountant, but her step had a new warmth and lightness. She began leading workshops on stress management and emotional resilience at her firm, sharing her journey and the techniques from her Resilience Toolkit that had helped her shift from worry to empowerment. Emma's transformation didn't stop there. She began volunteering at a local community center, leading financial literacy classes for underprivileged families. She found joy in helping others navigate their economic challenges, using her skills to empower them just as she had empowered herself. Her energy and enthusiasm were infectious, and soon, she was asked to join the board of a local nonprofit focused on mental health awareness—a cause she now felt deeply passionate about.

Through these experiences, Emma discovered a new sense of purpose. She realized that building emotional resilience wasn't just about managing her worries and fostering strength and support in her community. She became a mentor, a leader, and an advocate, using her story to inspire others to reclaim 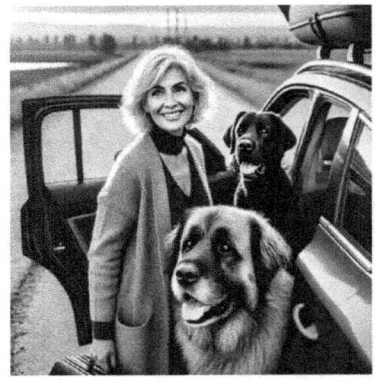 their lives from the grip of anxiety and fear. Over time, Emma found herself thriving in ways she hadn't imagined. Her relationship with her son blossomed as they bonded over shared experiences and new adventures. Seeing her transformation, her parents felt more at ease, knowing their daughter was equipped to handle whatever life threw at her. And Emma herself felt more fulfilled than ever, living a life filled with joy, connection, and purpose. Her Resilience Toolkit had become a powerful ally, guiding her toward a worry-free, empowered life. Emma's journey illustrates that even the most accomplished are not immune to the pitfalls of worry. But with the right tools and mindset, we can all build a life that's not just free from fear but filled with endless possibilities.

"To love oneself is the beginning of a lifelong romance."

— Oscar Wilde

Peter's Resilience in the Face of Job Loss

A 55-year-old manager, Peter had always been the rock in his professional and personal life. Known for his steady leadership and calm demeanor, he was the one colleagues turned to when things got tough. But when his company underwent a major restructuring and he suddenly lost his job, Peter found himself on shaky ground for the first time in decades. To make matters worse, amid this career upheaval, his wife announced she wanted a divorce. The double blow hit him hard, and he felt like the ground had been pulled out from under him.

Worry quickly consumed Peter—about his financial security, career prospects, ability to support his family, and the loss of his marriage. He lay awake at night, staring at the ceiling, a storm of fear and uncertainty swirling in his mind. He felt overwhelmed and unprepared for such a sudden and profound change. For a moment, everything he had worked for seemed unraveling. But Peter, ever the optimist, decided that he wouldn't let this be the end of his story. Instead of letting these setbacks paralyze him, he chose to build himself back up, stronger than before.

Peter knew he needed to shift his mindset. He began attending a local support group for job seekers. At first, he was hesitant. Sharing his fears and failures with strangers felt daunting, but he quickly found solace in the camaraderie and support of others facing similar challenges. Hearing their stories, he realized he was not alone. Many were in the same boat, navigating uncertainty and searching for new beginnings. The group became a lifeline, a source of encouragement and inspiration.

Determined to manage his stress healthily, Peter took up mindfulness meditation. Each morning, he would sit quietly, focusing on his breath, letting go of the worries that had weighed him down. At first, his mind raced, but he found a sense of calm and clarity over time. He began to understand that while he couldn't control everything that had happened, he could control how he responded. This realization was powerful. It started a new chapter where Peter focused on growth rather than fear.

Peter embraced a growth mindset and saw his career setback as an unexpected opportunity to explore new paths. He asked himself questions he hadn't considered in years: What did he truly enjoy? What kind of work would bring him fulfillment? He realized he had spent so much time climbing the corporate ladder that he had never thought about what made him happy.

With this newfound perspective, Peter decided to step out of his comfort zone. He began volunteering at a local non-profit, using his management skills to help with their operations. He found joy in the work, helping to streamline their processes and mentoring younger staff. This experience filled his time and renewed his sense of purpose and connection. He found that giving back was not just a way to keep busy but a way to heal and grow. It allowed him to see his value beyond a job title or salary.

As Peter continued this path of self-discovery, he also started to reconnect with himself in ways he hadn't before. He dusted off his old guitar and began playing again, a hobby he had abandoned years ago. He joined a community band, where he found joy in playing music with others. He even tried his hand at painting, something he'd never done before, finding it surprisingly therapeutic. He rediscovered passions and interests buried under years of routine and responsibility.

Over the months, Peter's resilience grew. He became a beacon of positivity, not just for himself but for those around him. His friends and family noticed the change in him. He was no longer the man who had lost his job and his marriage. He was Peter, the guy who could take whatever life threw at him and turn it into something beautiful. His optimism was contagious, and people were drawn to his newfound zest for life.

Eventually, Peter found a new job, managing a large dog rescue, which aligned with his values and provided greater fulfillment than his previous role. It wasn't just a job but a place where he could make a real impact. They appreciated his skills and experience, and he continued to grow. He realized that this unexpected detour had led him to a place he might never have found otherwise, where he could thrive.

Through it all, Peter learned that building emotional resilience wasn't just about surviving challenges; it was about embracing them, finding new opportunities for growth and meaning, and allowing oneself to be transformed by the journey. His story is a powerful

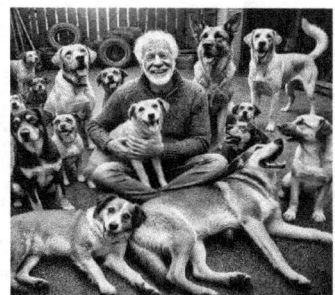

reminder that even in the face of life's greatest adversities, there is always a chance to rise, rebuild, and find a new path filled with purpose and joy. Peter emerged from his struggles not just as a survivor but as a dynamic, vibrant version of himself, ready to embrace whatever came next with an open heart and a hopeful spirit.

"Let go of the worries that weigh you down and focus on what lights you up. When you pursue what you love, you'll find that the things you used to fear no longer have power over you."

—Joanne Harvey

Chapter 7

Developing Healthy Habits to Reduce Worry

The Connection Between Physical Health and Mental Well-being

Our physical health directly impacts our mental well-being. Regular exercise, a balanced diet, and adequate sleep are crucial for maintaining a healthy body and a calm mind. Healthy habits can reduce stress and worry by improving overall health and resilience.

Techniques for Building Healthy Habits

1. **Establishing a Consistent Sleep Routine**: Good sleep hygiene is a cornerstone of mental and emotional well-being, especially when managing worry and anxiety. Creating a consistent sleep 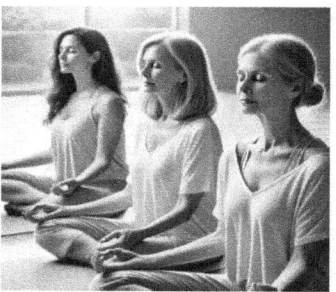 schedule is one of the most effective ways to promote restful, rejuvenating sleep. Start by setting a regular bedtime

and wake-up time, even on weekends, to help regulate your body's internal clock. Developing a calming bedtime routine can signal your body that it's time to wind down. This could include activities like reading a soothing book, practicing gentle stretches, or engaging in relaxation techniques like deep breathing or meditation. Reducing screen time before bed is essential because the blue light from phones, tablets, and computers can disrupt melatonin production, the hormone that regulates sleep. Consider creating a "digital sunset" by turning off screens at least an hour before bedtime, allowing your mind to transition smoothly into a restful state. Over time, these habits can help reduce sleep disturbances, improve the quality of your sleep, and provide a stronger foundation for managing worry and stress throughout the day. Good sleep hygiene not only aids in getting better sleep but also contributes to a clearer mind, a more balanced mood, and increased resilience against life's inevitable challenges.

2. **Incorporating Physical Activity into Daily Life:** Regular physical activity is a powerful tool for reducing stress, lifting your mood, and enhancing overall health. Exercise naturally releases endorphins—your body's feel-good hormones—which help counteract the effects of stress and anxiety. Beyond its immediate mental health benefits, regular physical activity improves sleep quality, increases energy levels, and fosters greater well-being. The key is finding an activity you genuinely enjoy and look forward to, a brisk walk in the park, a lively dance class, a calming yoga session, or an invigorating bike ride. Making physical activity a regular part of your routine doesn't have to feel like a chore; it can be a joyful, uplifting experience that you carve out time for each day. By dedicating even a small portion of your day to movement, you're nurturing your

body and reinforcing a positive, proactive approach to managing stress and enhancing mental resilience. Over time, this commitment to regular exercise can become a vital component of your resilience toolkit, helping you stay grounded, energized, and better equipped to handle whatever life throws your way.

3. **Nutrition Tips to Support Mental Health:** Nourishing your body with a balanced diet is essential for physical, emotional, and mental well-being. Consuming a variety of fruits, vegetables, whole grains, and lean proteins provides the necessary nutrients that fuel the brain, stabilize mood, and support overall cognitive function. Omega-3 fatty acids, found in foods like salmon, walnuts, and flaxseeds, have been shown to reduce symptoms of anxiety and depression. Meanwhile, antioxidant-rich foods like berries and leafy greens help fight inflammation and oxidative stress, which can harm brain health. It's equally important to avoid excessive intake of caffeine, sugar, and processed foods, as these can lead to energy crashes, exacerbate anxiety, and trigger mood swings. Maintaining steady blood sugar levels by eating regular, balanced meals and staying hydrated throughout the day can help keep your mind clear, your mood stable, and your energy consistent. Remember, nourishing your body with wholesome, nutrient-rich foods is a powerful act of self-care, laying the foundation for better mental health, greater resilience, and a more balanced, peaceful state of mind.

4. **Creating a Healthy Habit Plan**: Embarking on a journey to cultivate healthier habits is an act of self-love and compassion. Start by designing a personalized plan that gently integrates positive changes into your daily routine, focusing on sleep, exercise, and nutrition—critical pillars of

well-being. Set specific, measurable goals that feel both challenging and achievable; perhaps aim for a consistent bedtime, a daily walk, or adding more fruits and vegetables to your meals. Be kind to yourself as you establish these new habits; remember that progress, not perfection, is the goal. Keep a journal to track your progress, noting not just the physical milestones but also reflecting on subtle shifts in your mood, energy levels, and patterns of worry. Celebrate your successes, no matter how small, and approach any setbacks with understanding and grace. Over time, as these healthy habits take root, you'll likely notice a growing sense of calm, balance, and resilience. This journey is about nurturing yourself, finding joy, and honoring your commitment to a healthier, more vibrant life.

"Talk to yourself like you would to someone you love."

— Brené Brown

Michael's Transformation Through Healthy Habits

Michael was the kind of guy everyone in the neighborhood knew and loved. At 54, he had a heart as big as his smile, always ready to lend a hand or share a laugh. Known for his generosity, he was the type of person who'd literally give you the shirt off his back, no questions asked. Kids in the area often joke, "If you're ever in a jam, just find Michael. He's probably got a solution—and a sandwich!"

As a seasoned sales manager, Michael was no stranger to stress. His job was demanding, and he constantly worried about meeting targets, keeping up with the competition, and maintaining his health. The stress took a toll on him. He rarely found time to exercise, often grabbed meals on the go, and struggled with insomnia that left him dragging through his days. His doctor, concerned about his rising blood pressure and sleepless nights, strongly advised him to make some lifestyle changes. At first, Michael felt overwhelmed—how was he supposed to fit all this "healthy living" into an already packed schedule?

But Michael had a secret weapon: his love for cooking. He had always enjoyed whipping up meals, especially for others. Something about the sizzle of onions in a pan and the smell of fresh herbs made his heart feel lighter. So, he decided to use this passion as a starting point for his transformation.

He began experimenting with healthier recipes, swapping heavy ingredients for lighter, more nutritious options. Instead of his usual grab-and-go meals, he started preparing fresh, wholesome dishes in his kitchen. He had an idea as he became more invested in this new hobby. "Why not cook for others, too?" he thought. After all, he had plenty of neighbors who could use a good meal. And so, he started a little tradition: every Sunday, he'd cook up a storm and invite anyone hungry to swing by his place.

Word spread quickly. Michael's house became a hub of warmth and community, where no one was judged, and everyone was welcome. Neighbors began showing up with their dishes, and soon, these Sunday meals turned into a vibrant weekly potluck. But it wasn't just the food that drew people in—it was Michael's infectious positivity and genuine kindness. He had a knack for making everyone feel at home, whether they were an old friend or a new face.

Troubled kids in the neighborhood, who often found themselves on the streets with nowhere to go, started showing up, too. Michael welcomed them with open arms. He'd serve them a hot meal, listen to their stories, and offer encouragement. "You're always welcome here," he'd say. "Everyone needs a safe place to land." Before long, his home became a sanctuary, a haven where kids could escape their troubles, find a listening ear, and maybe even pick up a new recipe.

But Michael didn't stop there. He realized that to help others truly, he needed to take care of himself first. Inspired by his doctor's advice, he decided to overhaul his lifestyle. He started walking every morning, enjoying the crisp air and the quiet of the early hours. He joined a local yoga class, which became another community of support and friendship. He set a consistent sleep schedule, creating a calming bedtime routine that included reading, stretching, and meditation.

The changes didn't happen overnight, but Michael slowly noticed a difference. His anxiety levels started to drop, and the worries that once felt like a heavy weight on his shoulders seemed to lighten. He felt more energetic, focused, and—much to his surprise—happier. His newfound energy spilled over into his work, where he approached challenges with a clearer mind and a more positive outlook.

As Michael's physical and mental health improved, so did his outlook on life. He advocated for healthy living in his community, encouraging others to join him on his morning walks or to come for yoga. He started hosting cooking classes in his kitchen, teaching kids and young adults how to prepare nutritious, budget-friendly meals. His house was always bustling with activity—laughter, the clatter of dishes, the smell of good food, and the comforting hum of conversation.

His transformation didn't go unnoticed. Neighbors who once saw Michael as just "the nice guy down the street" now saw him as a beacon of positivity and resilience. He had taken what could have been a challenging period of his life and turned it into an opportunity for growth for himself and his entire community.

Michael's journey from stress and worry to health and happiness became a source of inspiration for everyone around him. He showed that building healthy habits wasn't just about living longer but about living better. It was about creating a life filled with joy, connection, and

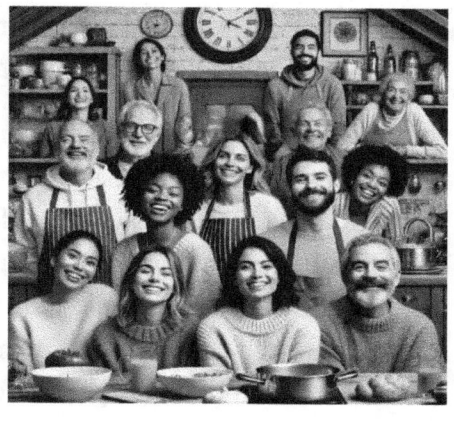

purpose. And in doing so, he reminded everyone that even in the face of life's challenges, there's always room for kindness, community, and a healthy meal shared with friends.

Laura's Journey to Health and Calm

Laura, a 48-year-old marketing executive, had established herself as a creative powerhouse in the boardroom and a champion worrier. She was known among friends and colleagues for anticipating every possible problem. "If there's a worry to be had, Laura's already worried about it," her coworkers would joke, affectionately dubbing her "Worry Queen." She wore the title with pride and frustration, knowing that her vigilance often served her well in navigating the unpredictable waters of corporate marketing. But at home, her worries took on a much heavier weight.

Her mother's battle with cancer and her father's rapidly progressing dementia were constant sources of concern. Laura's mind was always racing with "what-ifs"—what if her mother's treatment stopped working? What if her father wandered off and got lost again? What if she couldn't manage it all? On top of that, her job was as demanding as ever, and the combination of professional and personal pressures felt like juggling flaming torches while riding a unicycle on a tightrope.

Her life was a blur of back-to-back meetings, late-night phone calls with doctors, and sleepless nights worrying about her parents' health and her ability to keep up. Her fast-paced lifestyle left little room for healthy eating or exercise, adding to her stress. Laura's mind was a relentless ticker tape of anxiety, constantly cycling through a never-ending list of fears. She knew she was pushing herself too hard but didn't see any other way.

That all changed after a particularly grueling week. She had been up late every night working on a major campaign launch while juggling hospital visits and managing her father's care. Exhausted and running on fumes, Laura experienced a sharp, sudden pain in her chest that sent her to the emergency room. It was a minor health scare, but it scared her enough to realize something had to give. As she lay in the hospital bed, she couldn't help but think, "If I keep going like this, who's going to take care of my parents when I'm gone?" It was a sobering thought—a wake-up call she couldn't ignore.

Determined to change, Laura sought a wellness coach to help her find balance. Her coach, Maria, was kind but firm. "Laura," she said in their first meeting, "you're one of the top worriers I've ever met. But imagine what could happen if you used that energy for something positive?" Maria helped Laura craft a plan to fit her busy schedule without adding more stress. The goal wasn't to eliminate all worry—after all, some concerns are valid and necessary—but to find healthier ways to manage them.

They started with small, manageable steps. Laura began taking brisk walks during her lunch breaks, using the time to clear her head and soak in some much-needed sunshine. She signed up for a weekly cooking class, learning to prepare simple, nutritious meals that wouldn't take hours. This was a revelation for Laura; she discovered that cooking could be both a creative outlet and a form of self-care. She also began incorporating mindfulness practices into her daily routine, starting with a nightly wind-down routine that included turning off her devices, lighting a calming lavender-scented candle, and spending a few minutes meditating or reading.

At first, Laura's mind resisted. The "Worry Queen" in her wanted to jump right back into her usual cycle of stress and anxiety. But as she continued her new habits, she noticed subtle changes. Her body felt more substantial, her mind clearer. She was less reactive and more present at work and home. The constant knot of anxiety in her chest began to loosen, and she found herself laughing more and worrying less.

As her physical health improved, so did her mental state. She felt more energetic, less stressed, and more in control of her life. Her worries didn't vanish overnight, but they became more manageable. With her newfound resilience, she was better equipped to handle the inevitable challenges that came her way. When a particularly tough work deadline loomed, instead of panicking, she took a deep breath, mapped out a plan, and tackled it one step at a time. When her father had a difficult day, instead of spiraling into anxiety, she used her mindfulness techniques to stay calm and present, providing him with the comfort and support he needed.

Laura's transformation didn't go unnoticed. Her friends and colleagues marveled at the change. "You're still our Worry Queen," they teased, "but now you're like a Zen queen, too!" Laura would laugh, knowing they were right. She still had her moments of anxiety—after all, life was still full of challenges—but she had learned how to keep those worries from running her life.

Through her journey, Laura discovered that caring for herself wasn't a luxury but a necessity. It allowed her to show up fully for her parents, job, and, most importantly, herself. By prioritizing her well-being, she found a way to navigate her worries with grace and resilience. Laura's story is a testament to the power of small, intentional changes and their profound impact on reducing worry, enhancing resilience, and finding greater satisfaction and joy in life. She might still be known as the neighborhood's "Worry Queen," but now, she wore that title with a sense of humor and a balanced heart.

"You, as much as anybody in the entire universe, deserve your love and affection."

— Buddha

Use this space to jot down your thoughts, ideas, and any insights you gain as you work through the book. Let it be a place for reflection, breakthroughs, and practical takeaways that can help guide you toward a more peaceful mind.

_____
_____
_____
_____
_____
_____
_____
_____
_____
_____
_____
_____
_____
_____
_____
_____
_____
_____
_____

Chapter 8

Creating a Worry-Free Environment

The Role of Environment in Worry

Our surroundings significantly impact our mental state. A cluttered, chaotic environment can increase stress and worry, while a clean, organized space can promote calmness and clarity. Creating a worry-free environment involves decluttering, simplifying, and organizing physical and digital spaces.

Techniques to Declutter and Simplify Your Space

1. **Decluttering Tips for Your Home and Workspace:** Start small—focus on one area at a time, such as your desk or kitchen counter. Remove items that no longer serve a purpose or bring joy. Organize the remaining items in a way that promotes ease and efficiency.

2. **Creating a Calming, Worry-Free Zone:** Designate a specific area in your home or office as a worry-free zone. This space should be clutter-free and filled with items that

promote relaxation, such as plants, calming colors, or inspirational quotes.

3. **Minimizing Digital Distractions:** Digital clutter, such as an overflowing inbox or a disorganized desktop, can contribute to stress. Regularly delete unnecessary files, organize your emails, and limit time spent on social media.

Exercise: Conduct a "Worry Declutter"

Ask for help if you need to. Take it small at first. Identify areas in your home, workspace, or digital environment contributing to your worry. Set aside weekly time to declutter these areas and create a more peaceful, organized environment. Reflect on how these changes affect your mental state and worry levels.

Janet's Journey to a Worry-Free Environment

Janet was a happily married woman with a supportive wife and three overly attentive dogs who acted like her personal entourage. She adored her life, but there was one little hiccup—her house was a total disaster zone. Piles of papers teetered on every surface, books were stacked in precarious towers, and the amount of unused equipment collecting dust could probably be stocked in a small electronics store. Janet often worried that one rogue candle or an over-enthusiastic tail wag from one of the dogs could spark a fire. And she couldn't shake the fear that her wife might turn tomato-red with embarrassment if anyone dropped by unannounced and saw the state of their home.

At 69, Janet was a seasoned freelance writer with a knack for spinning words into magic, but her cluttered environment made her feel more like she was spinning in circles. Her home office looked like a cross between a library after an earthquake and an episode of "Hoarders." Her digital world was chaotic—endless emails, random files named "Final_Final_Version2," and social media notifications popping up like unwelcome guests at a party. She felt trapped in her cluttered surroundings, like a hamster on a wheel of worry and anxiety.

One day, after tripping over a stack of old magazines (which led to a dramatic fall that left her three dogs barking furiously, convinced a hitman had taken her out), Janet decided enough was enough. She'd recently read an article about the impact of a cluttered environment on mental health and realized it was time for a change. Her wife, ever the cheerleader, thought decluttering was a fantastic idea—especially since it meant she wouldn't have to keep creatively explaining their "lived-in" look to unexpected guests. They rolled up their sleeves and spent weekends diving into the chaos, sorting through piles, donating a mountain of unused items, and tossing out things they hadn't even realized they owned.

They approached it with humor and determination. As they unearthed long-lost items, they joked about finding the Ark of the Covenant under the stacks of paper. Janet found an old manuscript she had started in the '90s, much to her wife's amusement, titled "The Unfinished Novel," which now seemed like a perfect metaphor for the state of their home. They laughed so much that even the dogs seemed to catch the decluttering bug, enthusiastically chewing up some of Janet's old drafts. As Janet tackled her digital clutter, she unsubscribed from newsletters that had somehow become time travelers from 2003 and ruthlessly organized her digital files. She even put a limit on her social media time—after realizing she didn't need to be the first to know about every viral cat video (though the dogs strongly disagreed).

Within a few weeks, Janet noticed a significant shift in her mood and productivity. Her mind felt clearer, like someone had opened a window and let in fresh air. She was less prone to spiraling into worry, and her work became more focused and efficient. Her home, once a source of stress, now felt like a sanctuary. Creating a worry-free environment gave her a newfound sense of calm and focus, allowing her to enjoy her downtime without the constant buzz of anxiety in the background.

Feeling lighter and more liberated, Janet and her wife decided to add a fun new tradition to their routine: a weekly trip to the lake. It wasn't just for them—the dogs needed some fun after all their hard work of barking at boxes and shredding papers. These trips became a 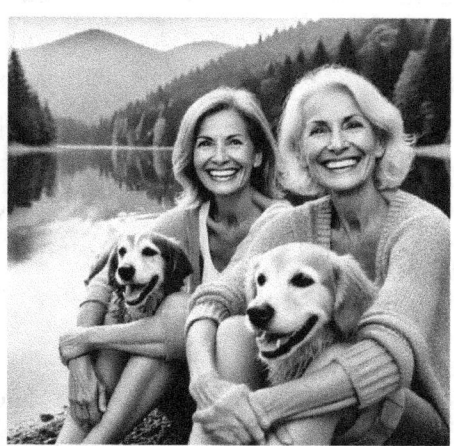 delightful escape, filled with laughter, splash fights, and doggy paddles. For Janet, life felt more balanced; her worries had quieted, and she discovered that decluttering could make room for more joy and spontaneity.

Samuel's Digital Declutter

Samuel, a 50-year-old IT specialist, had spent most of his life navigating the digital world with ease, helping others solve complex tech problems with the patience of a seasoned pro. Yet, Samuel was drowning in a sea of clutter regarding his digital space. His inbox was a nightmare of unread emails—some dating back years. His desktop was a chaotic mess of files and folders with cryptic names like "Report_Final_v2" and "VacationPics_2018_Final_Final," his social media notifications seemed to multiply faster than he could manage. The constant barrage of digital noise made him feel anxious and on edge, and he worried about missing something important or falling behind in his work.

Amidst all this digital chaos, Samuel found himself yearning for something more meaningful—he wanted to find a partner, someone to share his life with. He had recently started looking online for a potential Mrs. Samuel, browsing dating sites in the hopes of finding someone who might understand his quirks and share his dreams. But the irony wasn't lost on him: how could he present himself as organized and ready for a relationship when his digital life was in such disarray? The thought of a potential match catching a glimpse of his cluttered digital world made him cringe. His worries about digital clutter began to spill over into his personal life, affecting his self-confidence and readiness to find love.

Determined to regain control and create a digital space that reflected the person he wanted to be, Samuel decided to embark on a digital decluttering journey. He approached it with the same determination to do a challenging project. He started with his inbox, systematically going through each email, creating folders for important messages, and ruthlessly unsubscribing from newsletters and promotions he never read. As he cleared out the old emails, he felt a sense of relief wash over him. It was like he was clearing out old baggage, making room for new opportunities.

Next, Samuel tackled his desktop. He began categorizing files into specific folders, deleting duplicates, and archiving documents he no longer needed. He set up a routine for regular digital cleanups, realizing that just like a physical space, his digital environment required regular maintenance to stay organized and efficient. Finally, he took a hard look at his social media usage. Samuel decided to limit his time online, setting specific times of day to check his accounts and cutting back on the mindless scrolling that often left him feeling more disconnected. He even took a break from some platforms, realizing that real connections mattered more than online validation.

The result of this digital decluttering journey was transformative. Samuel felt a weight lift from his shoulders as his anxiety levels decreased. He was no longer overwhelmed by the constant barrage of notifications and digital noise. He found himself more focused, productive, and at peace with a more transparent, more organized digital space. His newfound mental clarity gave him the confidence to put himself out there, to be more open to the possibilities of finding love.

As Samuel navigated the world of online dating with his renewed sense of self, he discovered that the process wasn't nearly as daunting as he had once feared. He was more present in his conversations, more authentic in his interactions, and less worried about the what-ifs. Decluttering his digital environment profoundly impacted his mental clarity and overall sense of peace, allowing him to approach his personal and professional life with a fresh perspective. Samuel realized that sometimes, to find what you're genuinely looking for, you must start by clearing away what no longer serves you, making space for what truly matters.

"Clutter is not just the stuff on your floor; it's anything that stands between you and the life you want to be living."

– Peter Walsh

Chapter 9

The Power of Connection: Building Supportive Relationships

How Social Connections Influence Worry

Humans are social beings, and our relationships profoundly impact our mental and emotional well-being. Supportive, positive relationships can act as a buffer against worry and anxiety, while toxic or strained relationships can exacerbate these feelings. Building a network of supportive connections is crucial for reducing worry and fostering a sense of security and belonging.

Techniques for Building and Strengthening Support Networks

1. **Reaching out to Friends and Family:** Maintaining solid connections with friends and family is essential for emotional well-being, especially when facing worries or stress. Make a conscious effort to stay in regular contact with your loved ones through phone calls, video chats, or in-person visits. Sharing your worries with those you trust

lightens your emotional load and opens the door for empathy and support. It's a two-way street—being open about your struggles creates a safe space for others to share their concerns. This reciprocal sharing can deepen your relationships, fostering mutual understanding and connection.

Regularly reaching out doesn't have to mean lengthy conversations; sometimes, a quick text or a simple "thinking of you" message can strengthen bonds and provide comfort. These small gestures remind you and your loved ones that you're not alone and that someone cares. Additionally, actively listening when others share their worries can help shift your focus away from your anxieties, broadening your perspective and reinforcing the idea that everyone faces challenges. Open communication helps build a network of emotional support, alleviating feelings of isolation and promoting shared resilience.

Engaging in regular catchups or organizing small gatherings—whether a coffee date, a virtual game night, or a walk in the park—can help maintain these important connections. These moments of togetherness provide a sense of stability and belonging, making it easier to navigate difficult times. Remember, reaching out isn't just about seeking support; it's also about offering it. This act of giving and receiving compassion can strengthen your emotional foundation, reminding you that you are part of a caring, supportive community that can help weather any storm.

Lastly, don't hesitate to lean on your support network when things feel overwhelming. Friends and family can offer emotional comfort and practical advice or assistance. Knowing that you have people willing to listen and help can significantly reduce stress and improve your overall sense of security. By fostering these connections, you create a resilient safety net that can provide strength and comfort, helping you to feel more grounded, supported, and understood in times of worry or uncertainty.

2. **Joining Support Groups or Community Activities:** Engaging with support groups or participating in community activities can be a powerful way to build a sense of belonging and find comfort in shared experiences. Finding a group that aligns with your interests or reflects your current challenges can provide much-needed solidarity. Whether it's a local hobby group that meets regularly to discuss books, practice yoga, or enjoy gardening, or a spiritual community that gathers for meditation and reflection, these connections offer more than just companionship—they provide a safe space where you can express yourself freely without fear of judgment.

For those navigating more personal challenges, joining a support group specifically tailored to your experience— whether it's coping with grief, managing anxiety, dealing with chronic illness, or supporting a loved one through addiction—can be especially beneficial. These groups unite individuals who truly understand what you're going through because they've been there themselves. In these environments, you can share your feelings and experiences with people who get it, reducing the sense of isolation that often accompanies personal struggles. Hearing others' stories can also provide new perspectives and strategies, helping you feel less alone and more equipped to face challenges.

Community activities offer a unique opportunity to step out of your comfort zone and build new connections while engaging in something you enjoy. Whether it's joining a local sports league, participating in a volunteer organization, or taking a class on a topic that interests you, these activities provide a structured way to meet new people and develop a sense of community. The camaraderie built through shared goals and activities can significantly boost your mood and foster a sense of belonging and purpose. Engaging with your community in this way can also be a meaningful distraction from your worries, providing a healthy outlet for stress and anxiety.

Online support groups offer a flexible alternative for those who may find in-person groups challenging due to time constraints, location, or personal preference. Virtual communities can provide just as much support and connection as face-to-face interactions, often bringing together people from all over the world who share similar experiences or interests. Many online platforms offer forums, video meetings, and chat groups where you can engage at your own pace, participate in discussions, and build friendships without the pressure of a physical meeting. These digital communities can be especially comforting for those who feel more comfortable sharing their thoughts and feelings in a more anonymous setting or need support at unconventional hours.

By joining support groups or engaging in community activities, you create a network of support that extends beyond your immediate circle of friends and family. These connections can be invaluable, offering practical advice and emotional support. You may find comfort in knowing that you are part of a larger community, one that is willing to listen, share, and help you through whatever challenges you face. The simple act of being present with others, sharing a laugh, or engaging in meaningful conversation can be incredibly healing, reinforcing the idea that we are all in this together, each of us walking a path that, while unique, is also interwoven with the experiences of others.

Identify Your Support System

Write down the names of three people who provide positive support in your life. If you have one, this is still important. Commit to reaching out to them regularly, whether it's a weekly phone call, a monthly coffee date, or a simple text message. Reflect on how these connections help you manage worry and provide emotional support.

David's Transformation Through Community

A 56-year-old widower, David was once full of life, laughter, and endless optimism. But after losing his wife, his world felt like it had crumbled around him. The woman he had shared his life with for over three decades was gone, and he felt lost in a sea of sorrow. His days were consumed with worry—worry about his future, about his grown children who were trying to navigate their grief, and most of all, about his sanity. He feared he was losing his grip on reality, spiraling deeper into a dark hole of grief and anxiety. The house they once shared, filled with her laughter and warmth, now felt like an echo chamber of his fears and loneliness. His isolation only intensified his feelings of dread, leaving him to question whether he could ever find a way out of his despair.

One day, a neighbor stopped by as David sat on his porch, staring blankly at the garden his wife had lovingly tended. Sensing David's pain, the neighbor gently suggested he consider joining a local community church that offered a variety of support groups, including one specifically for grief. At first, David was hesitant.

The idea of opening up to strangers about his deepest, most personal pain felt daunting. He had always been a private man, keeping his struggles close to his chest. But something in his neighbor's kind eyes and reassuring words made him reconsider. With a mix of reluctance and desperation, David decided to try it. After all, what did he have to lose?

Walking into the church for the first time, David felt a knot of anxiety in his stomach. He wasn't sure what to expect and feared being judged or misunderstood. But to his surprise, he was greeted with warmth and genuine friendliness. The community welcomed him with open arms, offering smiles, handshakes, and a comforting sense of belonging that he hadn't felt in a long time. As he sat through the service, he felt a strange sense of calm beginning to wash over him. For the first time in months, he didn't feel completely alone. After the service, he heard about a weekly grief support group in a church's cozy meeting room. Hesitant but curious, David decided to attend the next session.

The support group was small, just a handful of people, each carrying their burden of loss. But there was an immediate sense of understanding and empathy in the room. As David listened to others share their stories—stories of lost spouses, parents, and children—he felt a sense of relief. Some people truly understood what he was going through and had walked similar paths of pain and heartache. When it was his turn to speak, he hesitated, unsure if he could find the right words. But as he began to talk about his wife, his fears, and his struggles, he felt a weightlifting from his chest. The group listened compassionately and offered words of support that felt genuine and heartfelt. For the first time, David didn't feel judged or pitied; he felt understood.

Over the weeks, David found himself looking forward to these meetings. He began to open up more, sharing not just his grief but also his fears about his mental health. He admitted to the group that he worried he was losing his mind and that the endless loop of sadness and anxiety was slowly unraveling him. But instead of recoiling, the group rallied around him, offering reassurance and practical advice. They shared their moments of doubt and fear, making David realize that his worries were not a sign of weakness but a natural part of the grieving process. These connections slowly began to heal the wounds in his heart, bringing light into the darkness that had settled over his life.

As time went on, David started to feel a shift within himself. He wasn't cured of his grief—he knew that loss would always be a part of him—but he began to feel more grounded, more capable of facing each day with a bit more hope. He formed friendships within the group that extended beyond the church walls. They began meeting for coffee, going on walks, and sharing meals. These simple acts of connection became a lifeline, helping him rediscover the joy of companionship and the comfort of shared experiences. David even began volunteering at the community center, helping organize events and lend a hand wherever possible. Giving back gave him a renewed sense of purpose, something he hadn't felt in a long time.

Through these new relationships and his growing involvement in the community, David realized that he wasn't alone in his struggles. His sense of isolation began to fade, replaced by a feeling of belonging and acceptance. The constant worry that had once paralyzed him slowly loosened its grip. By connecting with others who understood his journey, David found strength in vulnerability and discovered that there could be healing and hope even in the depths of grief. The community he once feared would judge him became a powerful source of comfort, reminding him that while grief was a heavy burden, he didn't have to carry it alone. David's journey through the darkness led him to a place of light, where friendship, faith, and community became the pillars of his resilience, guiding him back to a life where joy and sorrow could coexist and where love, even in loss, remained the greatest gift. David knew he didn't need to worry anymore; he had friends and support to help him.

Julia's Journey to Finding Support

Julia, a 53-year-old graphic designer, had always been a bit of a loner. She thrived in the quiet comfort of her routines, finding solace in the predictability of her daily life. Her work kept her busy, and she took pride in her creativity, often losing herself in intricate design projects late into the night. Solitude was her safe space; it allowed her to recharge and process her thoughts without the outside world's distractions. However, Julia's carefully constructed world unraveled when her only daughter left for college. The house that once buzzed with life and laughter now felt unbearably quiet, and the silence seemed to amplify her worries.

Julia was spiraling into a cycle of worry, consumed by thoughts about her daughter's safety and future. Every news report about campus incidents or economic uncertainties made her panic. She worried endlessly: Was her daughter eating well? Was she making good choices? Did she have friends to lean on, or did she feel as lost and lonely as Julia? The empty nest seemed to echo with these fears, each room a reminder of her daughter's absence and the life Julia had built around her. The worry weighed heavily on her, making her feel more isolated than ever.

Concerned about her sister, Julia's younger sister suggested she join a local book club. "It's a great way to get out of the house," she said gently, "and you'll meet people who understand what you're going through." At first, Julia was resistant. The idea of sharing her worries with strangers, even over something as innocuous as a book discussion, felt daunting. But the silence of her empty home and her sister's encouragement eventually nudged her to try it. "What do I have to lose?" she thought, mustering the courage to attend her first meeting.

To her surprise, the book club was filled with warm, understanding women who welcomed her with open arms. They were a mix of ages and backgrounds, each with their own stories and struggles. Over cups of tea and discussions about novels, Julia opened up in ways she hadn't expected. She learned that many other women were also grappling with life changes—some were adjusting to retirement, others were managing health concerns, and a few, like Julia, were navigating the emotional terrain of an empty nest. There was an immediate bond, a shared understanding that comforted her in a way she hadn't felt in a long time.

As the months passed, Julia began looking forward to their meetings. She laughed more, her worries momentarily forgotten in the warmth of the group's camaraderie. The club wasn't just about books—it became a space where she could share her fears without judgment and hear the reassuring voices of those who had been through similar experiences. These gatherings sparked something in Julia, a reminder of the joys of connection she had once pushed aside. She even began meeting with some members for coffee outside the book club, enjoying the simple pleasure of companionship and conversation.

Through these newfound friendships, Julia's anxiety about her daughter began to ease. While valid, she realized that her worries were not unique or insurmountable. She wasn't alone in her fears; talking about them made them feel less overwhelming. She started to see her daughter's departure not as an ending but as a new chapter for both. Her daughter was experiencing life, learning, and growing, and Julia could do the same. Inspired by her new friends, she took a watercolor painting class, rekindling an old passion she had set aside when her daughter was young. She found joy in the creative process, learning something new, and in the company of others who shared her interests.

Julia's journey through her loneliness and worry illustrates the transformative power of supportive relationships. By opening herself up to new experiences and connections, she discovered a community that alleviated her fears and fostered a sense of belonging and security she hadn't realized she was missing. The book club became more than just a hobby—it became a lifeline, helping her navigate this new stage of her life with a newfound sense of confidence and hope. Julia learned that while change is inevitable and sometimes scary, it can lead to beautiful new beginnings, especially when shared with others who understand.

"Stop worrying about the potholes in the road and enjoy the journey."

— Babs Hoffman

Use this space to jot down your thoughts, ideas, and any insights you gain as you work through the book. Let it be a place for reflection, breakthroughs, and practical takeaways that can help guide you toward a more peaceful mind.

Chapter 10

Living a Worry-Free Life

Integrating Worry-Free Practices into Daily Life

Living a worry-free life doesn't mean never experiencing worry again; it means learning to manage worry in a way that doesn't control or define your life. Integrating the practices and techniques you've learned throughout this book into your daily routine is vital to sustaining a worry-free mindset.

Creating a Personal Worry-Free Action Plan

Develop a personalized action plan that includes daily, weekly, and monthly practices to help you maintain a worry-free life. This might consist of mindfulness exercises, regular physical activity, maintaining supportive relationships, and setting aside time for self-reflection and gratitude.

Continuing to cultivate a worry-free mindset requires ongoing effort and self-awareness. It's important to be patient with yourself and recognize that setbacks are a normal part of the process. When worry creeps back in, use the techniques you've learned to manage it and refocus your imagination on positive, constructive outcomes.

Exercise: Develop a Worry-Free Action Plan

Create a written action plan tailored to your specific needs and lifestyle. Include your chosen daily, weekly, and monthly practices, and set realistic goals for incorporating these into your routine. Revisit and revise this plan regularly to ensure it continues to meet your needs and supports your journey toward a worry-free life.

Maria's Ongoing Journey to a Worry-Free Life

Maria, a 58-year-old physician assistant (PA), is no stranger to hard work. She lives in a bustling household spanning three generations: her demented grandmother, who often wanders around the house naked in confusion; her alcoholic, mildly demented parents, who require constant attention; and herself, the youngest in the family but shouldering the heaviest burdens. Her seven siblings, scattered across the city, rarely stop by to help. They're always too busy, distant, or absorbed in their lives to lend a hand. This leaves Maria feeling overwhelmed and utterly alone in her responsibilities.

Her family's needs feel crushing, and her mind constantly worries. She worries about her grandmother's safety—what if she wanders out of the house again? She worries about her mother's diabetes—how much longer can her body withstand the strain of diabetes and alcohol? She worries about her father's erratic moods, swinging wildly between despair and anger. He never was an easy man. And beneath all these immediate concerns, a deeper worry gnaws at her: Will she ever find a life companion with so much on her plate?

How can she meet someone when her life is consumed by caregiving and managing the chaos at home?

Maria's worries are compounded by her approaching retirement from her job as a PA. She has dedicated decades to caring for others at work and home, and now the prospect of retirement brings anxieties. She frets over her financial security—will she have enough to support herself and her family? She worries about her health, knowing the toll that years of stress have taken on her body. Most of all, she worries about finding a purpose outside her caregiving role. She wonders if she will ever have time to live for herself or if she is destined always to be the one holding everyone else together.

Feeling trapped and desperate for change, Maria picks up a book on living a worry-free life. She's initially skeptical—what can a book teach her about dealing with her unique situation? But as she reads through the pages, something resonates with her. She realizes that while she can't control her family's behavior or circumstances, she can control how she responds to them. Inspired, Maria creates a personal action plan to help her manage her worries and reclaim peace.

She starts with a daily mindfulness practice, finding solace in the quiet reflection it provides. Every morning, she sets aside a few minutes to breathe deeply and focus on the present, letting go of the endless "what ifs" that plague her mind. She also joins a walking group in her community, realizing that she needs more than just solitude—she needs connection and physical activity to break the cycle of worry. The group walks become a cherished part of her routine, offering exercise and a chance to connect with others who understand the importance of regular exercise.

Maria begins a gratitude journal, writing down five things she is grateful for at the end of the day. At first, it's difficult; her mind is used to worrying about the negative. Slowly, she starts to notice the small moments of joy—a kind word from a neighbor, the way the morning sun filters through the kitchen window, the smell of a pine tree, and the rare lucid moments with her grandmother that bring a smile to her face. These small acknowledgments of gratitude shift her perspective, making her feel more grounded and less anxious about the future.

Determined to create a more peaceful environment, Maria decluttered her home, turning it from a chaotic mess into a sanctuary of calm. She cleared out old, unused items, organized her spaces, and created a cozy corner where she could retreat when she needed a moment to herself. This physical decluttering mirrors her emotional decluttering; as her home became more orderly, so did her mind. She finds that having a clean, serene space helps her cope better with the daily demands of caregiving.

Through these practices, Maria begins to view her worries in a new light. Instead of seeing them as a burden, she sees them as signals to pause and refocus her energy. She learns to use her imagination not for conjuring worst-case scenarios but for envisioning more positive, constructive outcomes. She starts to dream again—about traveling, perhaps meeting a kindred spirit who understands her journey and finding fulfillment in her own right. She realizes that while she has many responsibilities, they do not have to define her entirely.

Maria's ongoing journey to a worry-free life becomes a testament to the power of intention, mindfulness, and self-care. She learns that while she can't change her past or control her family's behavior, she can change how she responds to her circumstances. By nurturing herself and seeking joy in the small moments, Maria finds a new sense of hope and possibility. Her life is still full of challenges, but she faces them with a renewed sense of strength and a belief that she deserves to live fully and joyfully.

George's Road to Rediscover His Life

George, a 60-year-old retired lawyer, finds retirement much more challenging than he ever imagined. What he thought would be a time of relaxation and freedom became filled with worry. He frets about his purpose now that he's no longer working, questions whether his finances will hold up over time, and worries about his health as he ages. Even his old dog and cat are a source of concern—he's constantly anxious that they're not getting the proper nutrition. George has always believed that worrying somehow keeps problems at bay, as if his constant vigilance could prevent anything from going wrong.

But as the days go by, George realizes this endless worrying is taking a toll on his happiness. He feels stuck, restless, and more anxious than ever. Determined not to let worry steal his retirement, he decides to make a change. He comes up with a "Worry-Free Action Plan," a personal roadmap to help him navigate this new chapter of his life with a bit more peace and a lot less anxiety. First, he signed up to volunteer at a local community center to use his skills to help others and connect with people meaningfully. Next, he incorporates daily meditation into his routine, hoping to find inner calm and break the habit of overthinking. He also commits to regular exercise, believing that staying active will help keep his mind and body healthy.

In a burst of inspiration, George finally picks up painting— something he's always wanted to try but never had time for during his busy career. He buys a set of paints and canvases and sets up a small studio in his spare room. At first, he feels awkward, not quite knowing where to start, but soon, he finds himself getting lost in the colors and textures, feeling a sense of freedom he hasn't felt in years.

George begins to feel a shift as he throws himself into these new activities. His worries don't disappear completely—he still has moments of anxiety, especially when he thinks about the future or hears about the health scares of dear friends. But now, instead of letting these worries control him, he uses them as reminders to engage more fully in the present, to focus on the things that bring him joy and fulfillment. Volunteering gives him a sense of purpose, painting sparks his creativity, and meditation helps him find peace amidst the chaos.

George's journey shows that it's never too late to redefine what life can be, even after a long career and years of ingrained habits. By taking proactive steps and embracing new passions, he finds a way to create a future that isn't dominated by worry but filled with joy, purpose, and new 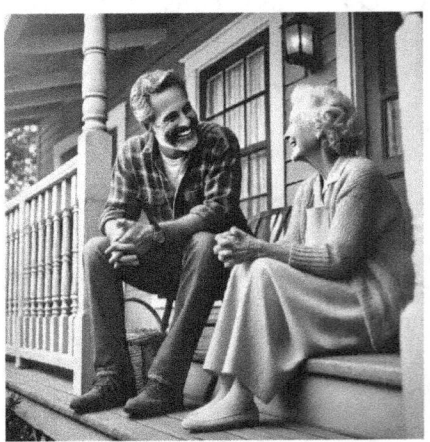 adventures. In doing so, he learns that sometimes, the best way to keep problems at bay is not to worry about them incessantly but to live each day with good intentions and an open heart.

Use this space to jot down your thoughts, ideas, and any insights you gain as you work through the book. Let it be a place for reflection, breakthroughs, and practical takeaways that can help guide you toward a more peaceful mind.

Chapter 11

Cultivating a Positive Mindset Through Affirmations and Visualizations

The Power of Positive Thinking

A positive mindset doesn't mean ignoring life's challenges or pretending everything is perfect. Instead, it's about approaching challenges with hope and possibility rather than fear and defeat. Affirmations and visualizations are powerful tools to cultivate a positive mindset, helping to reprogram negative thought patterns and reinforce a more optimistic outlook.

Techniques for Creating Effective Affirmations

1. Keep Affirmations Simple and Specific: Make sure your affirmations are clear and focused on a specific outcome or feeling. For example, instead of saying, "I want to be happy," try, "I am embracing joy and peace in my daily life."

Other examples include:

- "I am confident in my ability to handle whatever comes my way."

- "I am nourishing my body and mind with healthy choices."

- "I am deserving of love, support, and kindness from myself and others."

- "I am open to new opportunities and trust in the process of life."

- "I am releasing worry and welcoming calm and clarity into my life."

These affirmations focus on specific states of mind or goals, making them powerful tools for positive change.

2. Use Present Tense: Phrase your affirmations in the present tense as if they are already true. This helps your subconscious mind accept them as reality. For instance, "I am confident and capable in my work" rather than "I will be confident." Other examples include:

- "I am calm and centered, regardless of external circumstances."

- "I am attracting positive energy and opportunities into my life."

- "I am grateful for all I have and all that is coming my way."

- "I am strong, resilient, and able to overcome any challenge."

- "I am living a life filled with purpose and passion."

Using present-tense affirmations reinforces the belief that these positive states already exist in one's life, making them more effective in shaping one's mindset and behavior.

3. Focus on Positive Language: Avoid negative words or phrasing. Instead of saying, "I am not worried," use a positive framing like, "I am calm and confident." Other examples include:

- "I am healthy and vibrant, filled with energy each day."

- "I am surrounded by love and positivity in all areas of my life."

- "I am at peace with my past and excited for my future."

- "I am embracing change as a natural and positive part of life."

- "I am thriving and growing in all aspects of my life."

    By focusing on positive language, these affirmations help reinforce a constructive mindset and encourage a more optimistic outlook.

Daily Affirmation Practice

Write down three affirmations that resonate with you. Repeat them aloud each morning and evening for at least 21 days. Notice any shifts in your mindset or feelings as you practice. Keep a journal to track your progress and reflect on your worry patterns or changes in your emotional state.

Techniques for Effective Visualization

1. **Create a Relaxing Environment:** Find a quiet, comfortable place where you won't be disturbed. Close your eyes and take a few deep breaths to relax.

2. **Visualize in Detail**: To create a powerful and effective visualization, immerse yourself fully in the scene by engaging all your senses. Choose a setting that brings you peace, joy, or a sense of freedom—perhaps a favorite natural place, like a tranquil forest, a sunlit beach, or a serene mountain retreat. Imagine yourself there, allowing every detail to come alive in your mind.

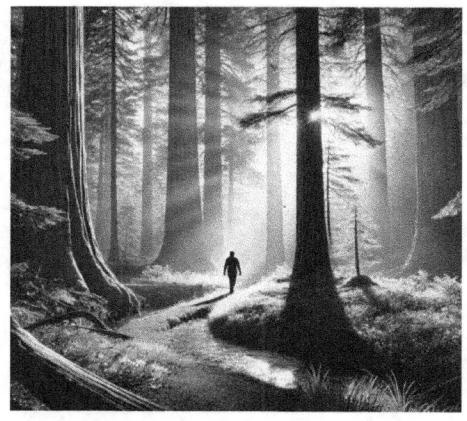

Picture yourself in the wilderness, surrounded by towering trees and gentle leaves rustling in the breeze. The sunlight filters through the canopy above, casting dappled patterns on the forest floor. You feel the soft crunch of pine needles underfoot as you walk along a winding path. The air is fresh and cool, filled with the earthy scent of moss and wildflowers. In the distance, you hear the melodic chirping of birds and the faint trickle of a nearby stream. As you breathe in deeply, the crisp, clean air fills your lungs, refreshing your body and calming your mind.

Or perhaps you visualize yourself swimming in the ocean, where the saltwater feels warm and buoyant against your skin. The sun glistens on the waves, and you hear the rhythmic sound

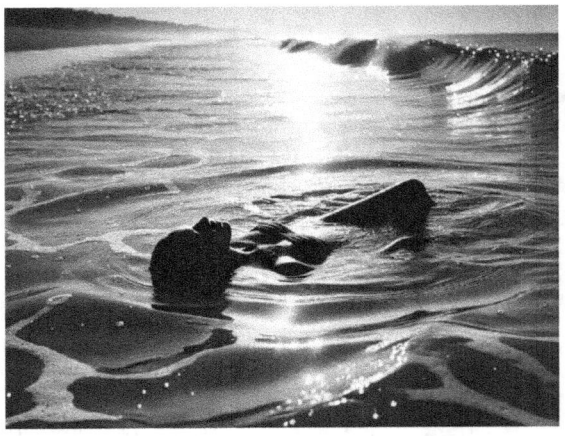

of the surf crashing gently on the shore. The taste of salt lingers on your lips, and you feel the cool, refreshing water enveloping you as you move effortlessly through it. You float on your back, feeling the sun's warmth on your face and the soothing sensation of the water supporting you, carrying away all your worries. The distant calls of seagulls mix with the whisper of the wind, creating a symphony of natural sounds that lull you into a state of deep relaxation.

If your favorite place is a cozy mountain cabin, imagine sitting on a wooden porch with a warm cup of tea in your hands. You hear the crackle of a fire inside, the soft whistle of the wind through the pine trees, and the distant call of an eagle

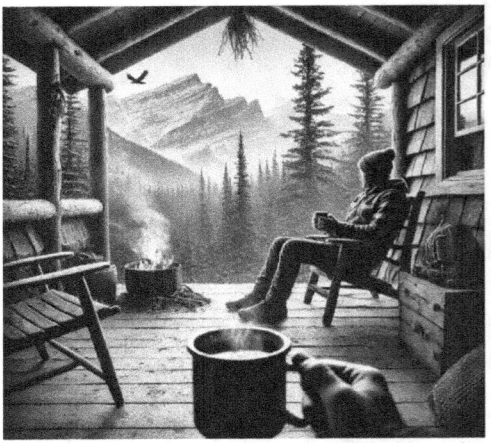

soaring high above. The scent of pine and woodsmoke fills the air, and you can taste the comforting warmth of the tea on your tongue. The view before you is breathtaking: snow-capped peaks under a clear blue sky, with a valley below that stretches out in an endless carpet of greenery. You feel the chair's solid wood beneath you, grounding you in the moment, as a gentle breeze caresses your face.

By visualizing these scenes with as much detail as possible—seeing the vibrant colors, hearing the specific sounds, feeling the textures and temperatures, smelling the distinct scents, and even tasting the elements present—you create a powerful mental experience. This detailed visualization is not just a mental exercise but a tool that empowers you to take control of your emotional well-being. It's a powerful technique that helps your mind and body relax like you are in that serene place, allowing you to escape daily stresses and bring a sense of calm, clarity, and renewal. The more vivid and sensory-rich your visualization, the more effectively it can transport you to a place of peace, enhancing your emotional well-being and helping you manage anxiety and worry.

1. **Focus on Positive Emotions:** As you visualize, immerse yourself in the positive emotions associated with the desired outcome. These positive emotions are not just a pleasant side effect of your visualization but the fuel that drives you toward your goal. Feel the deep fulfillment, warmth, and positivity of achieving your goal. Here are five more positive emotions you could focus on:

2. **Gratitude:** Feel a profound gratitude for all the steps that have led you to this moment. Appreciate the journey, the lessons learned, and the support from those around you. Allow this gratitude to fill your heart, enhancing your well-being and connection.

3. **Relief:** Experience relief as you visualize overcoming challenges or obstacles. Imagine the weight lifted off your shoulders and the sense of freedom that comes from knowing you have successfully navigated a difficult situation.

4. **Pride:** Embrace the feeling of pride in your accomplishments, no matter how big or small. Recognize the hard work, dedication, and resilience it took to reach your goal. Allow yourself to feel proud of your achievements and the person you've become.

5. **Contentment:** Feel a deep sense of contentment and satisfaction with where you are and what you have achieved. Visualize yourself at peace with your surroundings, feeling whole and complete in the present moment, without any desire for anything more.

6. **Empowerment:** Focus on the emotion of empowerment, feeling strong, capable, and in control of your life. Imagine making decisions with confidence and clarity, trusting your ability to shape your future and achieve your dreams.

Concentrating on these positive emotions during your visualization reinforces a positive mindset. It creates a powerful emotional state that can help you stay motivated, overcome challenges, and move closer to your goals with confidence and joy.

Erin's Transformation Through Affirmations

Erin is a dedicated and highly competent social worker known for her empathy, attention to detail, and unwavering commitment to her clients. She spends her days navigating complex cases, often involving children in dire situations who need her help. Her colleagues admire her ability to remain calm under pressure and her compassion for the families she works with. But beneath her professional demeanor, Erin is a constant worrier. She lives with a gnawing fear that her boss might fire her at any moment, even though she consistently performs well and receives positive feedback. This fear isn't grounded in reality, but it's always there, a persistent shadow that darkens her days.

Erin's anxiety doesn't stay at the office; it follows her home, where it takes on new forms. She worries about her three children—a three-year-old boy, a four-year-old daughter, and a baby boy. Her husband works the night shift, so they hardly get to talk about her concerns or share the burdens of daily life. She feels the world's weight on her shoulders, responsible for everything from keeping the household running to ensuring her children are happy and safe. She often feels overwhelmed, constantly juggling her demanding job, her duties as a mother, and the creeping doubts that make her question her worth and ability.

The stress of her job compounds her worries. Every day, Erin deals with cases that break her heart—children who are neglected, abused, or otherwise harmed by the very people who are supposed to care for them. She knows that removing a child from a harmful environment is sometimes the best and only option, but it doesn't make the decision any easier. She agonizes over each case, wondering if there was something more she could have done, some way to keep the family together. She feels a deep sorrow for the children she has to remove from their parents, knowing the trauma and confusion they must feel. These thoughts haunt her at night when the house is quiet and her husband is working. She lies awake, staring at the ceiling, worrying about the children she couldn't save and the families that were torn apart.

The constant worry takes its toll. Erin becomes increasingly irritable, snapping at her kids over minor things—spilled milk, a left-out toy, and a tantrum. She hates how she's been acting but feels like she's always on edge, her nerves frayed from the stress of trying to be everything to everyone. Sensing her tension, her children become more clingy, adding to her frustration. She feels guilty for her short temper and worries she's not being the mother they need. The guilt piles on top of her existing worries, creating a cycle of anxiety and self-doubt that seems impossible to break.

With her husband working nights, Erin doesn't have a chance to talk through her concerns. Their conversations are often rushed—quick phone calls or messages in passing when he comes home in the early morning hours, tired and needing sleep. She feels isolated in her struggles, unable to share the emotional burden with the one person she trusts most. The lack of communication strains their relationship, adding another layer of worry to Erin's already overloaded mind. She fears they're drifting apart but doesn't know how to reach out when her concerns consume her.

One day, after a particularly tough case involving a young child removed from a home with a violent parent, Erin reaches a breaking point. She finds herself crying in the bathroom at work, feeling utterly helpless and alone. Her boss, noticing her distress, gently approaches her later in the day. "Erin, I can see you're carrying a lot," she says softly. "You're doing an incredible job, but you don't have to do it alone. Have you considered talking to someone about what you're going through?"

Her boss's words stick with her, and Erin realizes she's been carrying her burdens in silence for far too long. She decides to seek help and reaches out to a therapist who specializes in working with social workers and other professionals dealing with secondary trauma. In therapy, Erin begins to unpack her fears, her guilt, and her constant worry. She learns that her feelings are normal and that feeling overwhelmed is okay. The therapist helps her develop strategies to manage her anxiety, encouraging her to set boundaries at work and to practice self-care.

Her transformation involves integrating positive affirmations into her daily routine, which her therapist suggests helps shift her mindset from fear and doubt to strength and self-compassion. Each morning, Erin starts her day with a few affirmations, speaking the affirmations aloud while looking in the mirror. "I am enough, just as I am," she tells herself, reminding herself that her worth isn't defined by her ability to fix every problem or save every child. "I am doing my best, and that is enough," she repeats, allowing herself to let go of the unrealistic expectations she places on herself.

Throughout the day, whenever she feels her anxiety rising, Erin silently recites affirmations like "I am loved, and I am loving." These words become a lifeline, grounding her in moments of doubt and reminding her to be kind to herself. She also adds affirmations that focus on her strengths, such as "I am a compassionate and skilled social worker who makes a difference" and "I am a loving mother who provides safety and love for my children." Over time, these positive statements begin to take root, slowly replacing worry and fear with a growing sense of confidence and self-assurance.

Erin also opens up more to her husband, finding moments in their busy schedules to share her feelings. They begin setting aside time for regular check-ins, even if it's just a few minutes each day. Her husband listens with patience and understanding, and Erin feels a weight lift off her shoulders as she shares her burdens. They work on finding ways to support each other better, recognizing that they're in this together, even if their schedules are challenging and designed for their kids.

At home, Erin begins practicing mindfulness and breathing exercises to calm her mind when her worries spiral. She also sets aside dedicated playtime with her children, allowing herself to be fully present in those moments, free from distractions and work pressures. These small changes make a big difference. She starts noticing a shift in her mood and interactions with her family. She becomes less irritable and more patient, finding joy in her children's laughter and learning to forgive herself for not being perfect.

Through these efforts and the power of her affirmations, Erin begins to find a new balance. She still worries it's her nature but no longer lets her fears control her. She realizes that being a good mother, a loving wife, and a dedicated social worker doesn't mean she has to be perfect. It means doing her best with what she has, accepting her limitations, and knowing when to ask for help. Her journey toward managing her worries and finding peace is ongoing, but each step she takes brings her closer to a life where she feels more in control, more connected, and more at ease with herself and the world around her.

Jason's Use of Visualization for Career Success

Jason, a 55-year-old graphic designer, often finds himself drowning in worry about his career future. The industry seems to change overnight with new technologies and trends, and Jason fears becoming obsolete, left behind by younger, more tech-savvy competitors. He spends countless nights tossing and turning, his mind racing with concerns about finding new clients and staying relevant in a rapidly evolving market. The constant worry gnaws at him, affecting his creativity and motivation. He feels stuck, like he's treading water in a sea of uncertainty.

One day, while scrolling through an online forum for creative professionals, Jason stumbles upon a discussion about visualization techniques. Intrigued, he reads about how imagining positive scenarios can help reduce anxiety and refocus the mind on achieving desired outcomes. Jason tries visualization to find a way out of his worry cycle. He begins each morning by closing his eyes and picturing his ideal work situation. He imagines himself confidently presenting his latest designs to a room full of satisfied clients. He sees their faces light up with admiration and hears their voices praising his creativity and skill. In his mind, he feels the warmth of their appreciation and the deep sense of fulfillment from knowing he's done a great job.

But as Jason continues practicing his visualizations, he decides to go even deeper, to a place that brings him true peace and joy— swimming in the warm ocean, surrounded by turtles and beautiful fish. Each day, he closes his eyes and takes a few deep breaths, letting go of the tension in his body. He imagines himself diving into crystal-clear, turquoise waters. The ocean is warm against his skin, enveloping him in a comforting embrace. As he swims, he can feel the gentle push and pull of the waves, the saltwater soothing his worries away. Around him, a school of vibrant, colorful fish darts playfully through the water, their scales shimmering in the sunlight that filters down from above.

Jason envisions himself gliding effortlessly through the water, his movements in perfect harmony with the rhythm of the sea. Nearby, a group of sea turtles swims gracefully alongside him, their slow, steady movements calming his mind. He reaches out to touch one of the turtles, feeling its shell's cool, smooth texture beneath his fingertips. The turtle turns its head slightly as if acknowledging him, and Jason feels a deep sense of connection and tranquility. He takes a moment to pause, floating on his back, feeling the sun's warmth on his face and the gentle caress of the ocean breeze. He listens to the soothing sounds of the waves and the distant calls of seabirds overhead.

As Jason practices this visualization daily, he notices a change within himself. The worries that once consumed him begin to lose their grip. The fears of becoming obsolete or failing to find new clients seem less daunting when he taps into the calm and confidence he feels while swimming in the ocean. His mind, once cluttered with anxiety, feels clearer and more focused. He realizes that he cannot control every aspect of his industry or the future but can control how he responds to these uncertainties. Instead of letting his fears paralyze him, he sees them as opportunities to grow and evolve.

Empowered by this newfound sense of peace and clarity, Jason decides to take more proactive steps in his career. He starts attending networking events with renewed purpose, eager to connect with potential clients and collaborators. He reaches out to old contacts and explores new avenues for showcasing his work. He even signed up for an online course to learn new design software, confident that he can adapt and thrive in a changing industry. With each step he takes, he draws from the calm and confidence he feels in his visualizations, carrying that sense of ease into his real-life interactions.

Over time, Jason notices a significant shift in his career. He has several new clients who are impressed with his work and his innovative approach. His anxiety about the future diminishes, replaced by excitement and anticipation for what's to come. Visualization has helped Jason transform his fears into a positive vision for his career, leading to real-world success. More importantly, it has taught him that even when the future is uncertain, he can always find a place of peace and strength within himself, like the warm ocean that washes away his worries and renews his spirit.

"It's a half an inch of water, and you think you're going to drown.

— John Prine

Chapter 12

The Journey Forward:
Sustaining a Worry-Free Life

Embracing Continuous Growth

A worry-free life is not a destination but a continuous journey of self-discovery and growth. It involves regularly assessing your mental and emotional state, learning from experiences, and adapting your strategies as needed. This chapter focuses on sustaining a worry-free mindset over the long term and embracing continuous personal development.

Strategies for Dealing with Setbacks

1. **Practice Self-Compassion:** Understand that setbacks are a natural part of life. Treat yourself with the same kindness and understanding that you would offer a friend facing a similar situation.

2. **Reflect and Learn:** Use setbacks as opportunities for growth. Reflect on what went wrong, what you learned from the experience, and how you can apply those lessons moving forward.

3. **Revisit Your Tools and Techniques:** When facing a setback, revisit the tools and techniques you've learned throughout this book. Use mindfulness, cognitive restructuring, and positive affirmations to navigate your feelings and regain control.

Reflection and Goal-setting

Set aside monthly time to reflect on your journey toward a worry-free life. Consider what has worked well, your challenges, and areas you'd like to improve. Set specific, achievable goals for the coming month, and plan how you will continue to practice and develop your worry-free techniques.

The Importance of Community and Support

Maintaining a worry-free mindset is more manageable when surrounded by supportive people who understand and encourage your journey. Consider joining a support group, finding a mentor, or staying connected with friends and family who uplift and inspire you.

Hannah's Continuous Journey of Growth

Hannah, a 57-year-old former horse trainer, has faced more than her share of challenges. She retired early due to health issues, leaving behind a career she loved and a cherished active lifestyle. Retirement, which she had hoped would be a time of relaxation and freedom, quickly became filled with worry about her future. With her health in decline, she struggled to maintain her independence and feared becoming a burden to her family. Her worries spiraled, making her feel increasingly isolated and anxious about what lay ahead.

Determined not to let these fears consume her, Hannah turned to the steps outlined in a book on managing worry. She started by journaling her fears, allowing herself to express her concerns on paper and examine them from a different perspective. She practiced mindfulness, focusing on the present moment rather than letting her mind wander to all the "what ifs" that plagued her thoughts. She also made a conscious effort to focus on the positive aspects of her life, reminding herself daily of what she was grateful for, like the support of her friends and the beauty of a sunrise. These practices helped her regain some sense of control, but setbacks came when her health declined further. She began to worry again about becoming a burden to her family, fearing that her needs would outweigh their capacity to care for her.

Just when despair threatened to take hold, Hannah decided to take action. She contacted her church community, hoping to find some guidance or support. Through this network, she discovered an over-55 community that offered affordable housing for people with low incomes and a range of supportive services for those with caregiving needs. Intrigued and hopeful, Hannah decided to explore this new possibility. The community offered precisely what she needed: a safe, supportive environment where she could maintain independence while receiving the required help.

Moving into the community was one of the best decisions Hannah ever made. From the moment she arrived, she felt welcomed and cared for. The staff were friendly and attentive, always ready to lend a hand with her daily needs, whether it was help with transportation to medical appointments or assistance with household chores. But more than the physical support, Hannah found herself surrounded by a group of lively, like-minded individuals who understood her struggles and shared her desire for companionship and fun.

Hannah quickly made new friends—people like her had experienced their share of life's ups and downs but were determined to make the most of their golden years. They found joy in simple pleasures: sharing meals, playing cards, and participating in organized community activities. Hannah was delighted to discover a range of options to keep her busy and entertained. She could choose between a day trip to the casino, where she could test her luck at the slot machines with her new pals, or a leisurely swim at the local lake, enjoying the cool water and warm sun on her skin.

Her worries shifted from fears about her future to lighthearted decisions about which fun activity to try next. She no longer felt like a burden; instead, she felt like a valued member of a vibrant community. The support from the staff and her new friends helped her regain a sense of independence and purpose. Her days were filled with laughter, friendship, and new experiences, a far cry from the lonely, anxious days she had faced.

The community also offered creative expression opportunities, which Hannah had missed since retiring from horse training. She signed up for an art class, where she discovered a talent for painting. She felt her worries fade with each brushstroke, replaced by a sense of calm and fulfillment. She even began to sell some of her artwork at the community's local craft fairs, earning some extra income and feeling proud of her accomplishments.

Through this journey, Hannah learned that her worries were not insurmountable. She realized she could still enjoy life and find new passions with proper support and a positive mindset, even with her health challenges. Her community became her anchor, where she could feel safe, supported, and connected. Her new friends became her second family, sharing her joys and helping her shoulder her burdens.

Instead of worrying about becoming a burden, Hannah focuses on each day's possibilities. She enthusiastically embraces her new life, thankful for the unexpected blessings that have come her way. Whether planning a spontaneous adventure with her friends or simply enjoying a quiet moment by the lake, Hannah knows she is exactly where she is meant to be. Her story is a testament to the power of community, resilience, and the enduring strength of the human spirit to find light even in the darkest of times.

Use this space to jot down your thoughts, ideas, and any insights you gain as you work through the book. Let it be a place for reflection, breakthroughs, and practical takeaways that can help guide you toward a more peaceful mind.

_____

_____

_____

_____

_____

_____

_____

_____

_____

_____

_____

_____

_____

_____

_____

_____

_____

_____

_____

_____

Conclusion: A Lifetime of Possibility

As I conclude this book, remember that worry wastes your imagination. You have the power to transform your thoughts and create a life filled with peace, joy, and creativity. Embrace each day with love, kindness, and curiosity, knowing you can handle whatever comes your way.

Your journey to a worry-free life is just beginning. May it be filled with growth, discovery, and endless possibilities. Always nurture yourself with compassion, surround yourself with supportive people, and use your imagination for positive, constructive purposes. Here's to a life free from worry and full of wonder!

And as you move forward, let love be your compass. Trust that you are exactly where you need to be and that everything unfolds in time. Approach each moment with an open heart, knowing that your worth is not defined by what you fear but by the courage you show in choosing joy over doubt.

May you always find the strength to release your worries and the wisdom to embrace the unknown with hope and optimism. Remember, you are never alone on this journey. You are loved, capable, and deserving of all the beauty life has to offer.

Here's to stepping boldly into a bright future filled with possibilities, love, and adventure, worry-free.

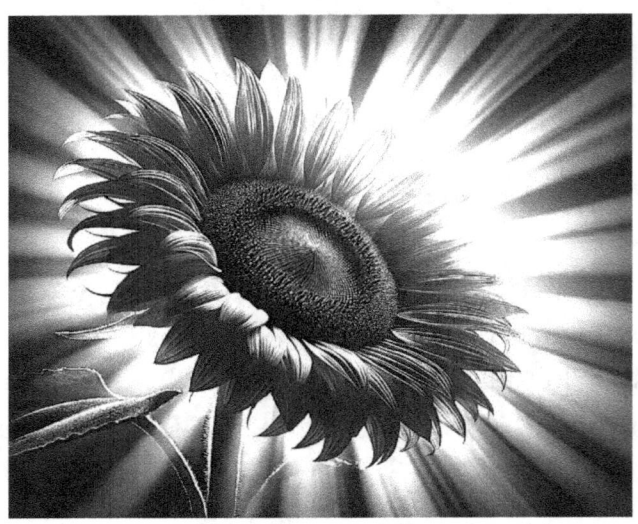

Resources and Continued Growth

To support you on your journey to a worry-free life, consider exploring the following resources:

1. Taren, A. A., et al. (2013). Mindfulness Meditation Training Alters Stress-Related Amygdala Resting State Functional Connectivity: A Randomized Controlled Trial. *Social Cognitive and Affective Neuroscience.*

2. Goyal, M., et al. (2014). Meditation Programs for Psychological Stress and Well-being: A Systematic Review and Meta-analysis. *JAMA Internal Medicine.*

3. Hofmann, S. G., et al. (2010). The Effect of Mindfulness-Based Therapy on Anxiety and Depression: A Meta-Analytic Review. *Journal of Consulting and Clinical Psychology.*

4. Hofmann, S. G., et al. (2012). Cognitive Behavioral Therapy for Anxiety Disorders: A Meta-Analysis of Randomized Placebo-Controlled Trials. *Psychiatric Clinics of North America.*

5. Goldin, P. R., et al. (2008). The Neural Bases of Emotion Regulation: Reappraisal and Suppression of Negative Emotion. *Biological Psychiatry*.

6. Barlow, D. H., et al. (2014). The Unified Protocol for Transdiagnostic Treatment of Emotional Disorders: A Randomized Controlled Trial. *Behavior Research and Therapy*.

7. Burns, David D. (2008). *When Panic Attacks: The New, Drug-Free Anxiety Therapy That Can Change Your Life.* Broadway Books.

8. Carlson, Richard, Ph.D. (1997). *Don't Sweat the Small Stuff...and It's All Small Stuff: Simple Ways to Keep the Little Things from Taking Over Your Life.* Hyperion.

9. Chodron, Pema. (2001). *The Places That Scare You: A Guide to Fearlessness in Difficult Times.* Shambhala Publications.

10. Leahy, Robert L., Ph.D. (2006). *The Worry Cure: Seven Steps to Stop Worry from Stopping You.* Harmony Books.

11. Bourne, Edmund J., Ph.D. (2011). *The Anxiety and Phobia Workbook.* New Harbinger Publications.

12. Orsillo, Susan M., & Roemer, Lizabeth. (2011). *The Mindful Way Through Anxiety: Break Free from Chronic Worry and Reclaim Your Life.* The Guilford Press.

13. Tolle, Eckhart. (2004). *The Power of Now: A Guide to Spiritual Enlightenment.* New World Library.

14. Clark, David A., & Beck, Aaron T. (2011). *The Anxiety and Worry Workbook: The Cognitive Behavioral Solution.* The Guilford Press.

15. Weekes, Claire. (1990). *Hope and Help for Your Nerves: End Anxiety Now.* Signet.

16. A classic self-help book that provides a compassionate approach to managing anxiety and worry.

17. Kabat-Zinn, Jon. (1990). *Full Catastrophe Living: Using the Wisdom of Your Body and Mind to Face Stress, Pain, and Illness.* Bantam Books.

Websites and Online Communities Focused on Mental Wellness

Here are some excellent websites that focus on mental wellness, offering resources, support, and information:

1. **Very Well Mind**: This website provides comprehensive information on mental health topics, including anxiety, depression, therapy options, mindfulness, self-improvement, and relationships. It's designed to help readers better understand mental health and find practical advice for healthier lives. You can explore various mental health conditions and find tips on managing stress and improving well-being.

2. **Mental Health America (MHA)**: MHA is a leading nonprofit organization promoting mental health and well-being. Its website offers a variety of resources, including mental health screening tools, educational materials, and advocacy opportunities. It is an excellent resource for anyone looking to understand mental health better and find support in their community.

Workshops and Support Groups for Stress Management and Emotional Resilience

1. **Mindfulness and Meditation Workshops:** A series of workshops that teach participants various mindfulness and meditation techniques to manage stress and reduce worry. These sessions could include guided meditation, breathing exercises, and mindful movement practices like yoga or Tai Chi.

2. **Cognitive Behavioral Therapy (CBT) Skills Training:** A workshop series that introduces the principles of CBT, focusing on identifying and challenging negative thoughts and developing healthier thinking patterns. This could include cognitive restructuring, thought records, and the ABCDE model.

3. **Emotional Resilience Building Groups:** Support groups that focus on developing emotional resilience through positive self-talk, growth mindset, and gratitude practices.

4. **Creative Visualization and Imagination Sessions:** Workshops that teach creative visualization techniques to help participants use their imagination constructively, focusing on positive outcomes and creative problem-solving rather than worry.

5. **Stress Management and Self-Care Retreats:** A weekend retreat focused on comprehensive stress management techniques, including physical activities (yoga, hiking), nutrition workshops, mindfulness practices, and sessions on emotional regulation.

6. **Activities:** Yoga and relaxation sessions, nutritional workshops, guided nature walks, group meditation

7. **Support Groups for Specific Worries:** These are targeted support groups for specific types of worries (Co-dependent, Al-Anon health-related worries, financial concerns, parenting worries). They provide a safe space for sharing experiences and learning coping strategies.

8. **Gratitude and Positive Psychology Workshops:** These workshops focus on cultivating gratitude and using positive psychology techniques to enhance emotional well-being and reduce stress.

9. **Book Clubs:** Align with chapters on positive affirmations, emotional resilience, and the importance of a positive mindset.

About the Author

Joanne Harvey, MSW, is a testament to embracing life with open arms. With a rich tapestry of experiences, Joanne's journey is marked by her unwavering commitment to reducing suffering and fostering resilience in others. She is the author of three impactful books, *"Worry is a Waste of Your Imagination: Strategies for A Worry Free Life," "Estranged Parent's Guide to Resilience: Achieving a Brighter Future"* and *"Sacred Light: True Stories of Legacy, Peace & Comfort in Hospice Care"*. Her writing offers a compassionate path toward healing, helping readers transform their lives from pain to peace and purpose.

Joanne's career spans diverse roles, each underscoring her dedication to service and well-being. She was a medical social worker in a large trauma hospital. She developed and ran a direct marketing company catering to women who fly fish. She managed a hay and registered cattle operation and served as a medical social worker for a local hospice. These varied experiences have given her unique insights into human behavior and the complexities of life, enabling her to connect deeply with her readers and clients.

Now, as a Progressive Emotional Freedoms Techniques Master and Certified Havening Practitioner, Joanne operates her private practice, providing guidance and support to individuals navigating life's challenges. Her compassionate approach, grounded in professional expertise and personal experience, helps clients and readers find resilience and joy, even in the face of adversity.

Living in the tranquil mountains of California with her husband, two spirited rescue dogs, two adventurous cats, and a dozen tiny chickens, Joanne continues to live by her philosophy of embracing life fully and fearlessly. She draws inspiration from her surroundings and remains dedicated to her passion for reducing suffering in all its forms. Whether she's writing, working with clients, or simply enjoying the beauty of her mountain home, Joanne Harvey embodies a spirit of hope, resilience, and love that shines through in everything she does.

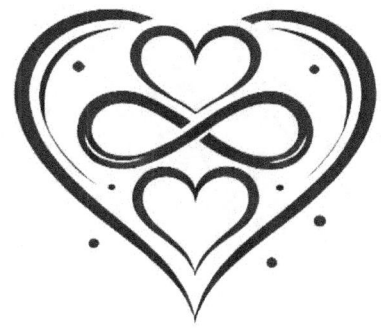

www.ingramcontent.com/pod-product-compliance
Lightning Source LLC
Chambersburg PA
CBHW082105140626
46553CB00018B/881